AF614705

METHODS IN MOLECULAR BIOLOGY™

Mouse Models of Innate Immunity

Methods and Protocols

Edited by

Irving C. Allen

Department of Biomedical Sciences and Pathobiology, Virginia-Maryland Regional College of Veterinary Medicine, Virginia Polytechnic Institute and State University, Blacksburg, VA, USA

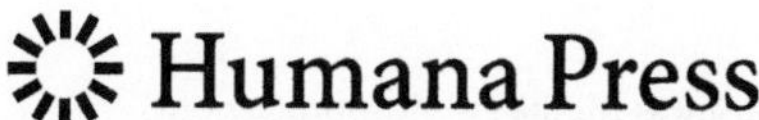

Editor
Irving C. Allen
Department of Biomedical Sciences and Pathobiology
Virginia-Maryland Regional College of Veterinary Medicine
Virginia Polytechnic Institute and State University
Blacksburg, VA, USA

ISSN 1064-3745 ISSN 1940-6029 (electronic)
ISBN 978-1-62703-480-7 ISBN 978-1-62703-481-4 (eBook)
DOI 10.1007/978-1-62703-481-4
Springer New York Heidelberg Dordrecht London

Library of Congress Control Number: 2013942305

Printed on acid-free paper

Humana Press is a brand of Springer
Springer is part of Springer Science+Business Media (www.springer.com)

Preface

Infectious diseases represent a significant global health threat. The rise of multidrug-resistant pathogens and the increased potential for the emergence of a catastrophic disease pandemic have ushered in a new era in immunology research, which has become more focused on understanding host–pathogen interactions. Throughout evolution, the immune system has shown an extraordinary ability to adapt and protect the host from pathogen invasion. The innate immune system represents a critical arm of the immune response by providing immediate and robust host defense. The cornerstone of the innate immune response is the diverse group of cells, including macrophages, neutrophils, and lymphocytes, that contribute to host defense through the recognition, isolation, and eradication of pathogens. These cells rely on an assortment of extracellular and intracellular pattern recognition receptors, which sense pathogen- or damage-associated molecular patterns, in order to initiate the hallmark molecular signaling cascades that are associated with innate immunity.

Biomedical research is driven by the desire to improve the health and welfare of human patients. However, human studies are often limited by ethical, logistical, and technical obstacles. In many cases, these obstacles can be difficult to overcome. In an effort to circumvent many of these limitations, researchers have turned to mice as either surrogate or complementary models for many human disease studies. The readily available assortment of genetically manipulated mouse strains provides researchers with powerful tools to dissect the complex interactions associated with the innate immune response and host defense. Advances in mouse genetics have occurred in parallel with human clinical studies, and, together, these strategies have significantly complemented our understanding of the disease processes associated with innate immunity.

Mouse Models of Innate Immunity: Methods and Protocols has assembled a diverse and highly regarded group of contributors with extensive experience in genetics, microbiology, immunology, and in vivo model systems. Similar to the other volumes in the *Methods in Molecular Biology* series, these contributors have provided detailed protocols for the design and execution of experiments to thoroughly evaluate critical elements associated with the host innate immune response. Emphasis has been placed on mouse models that accurately mimic clinically relevant disease processes in response to a variety of insults and pathogen exposures. The first half of this book focuses on methods that are essential for collecting and assessing various primary cells that are highly relevant to innate immunity. These ex vivo protocols provide simplified systems to evaluate hypotheses without many of the confounding issues that are often associated with the complexity of in vivo models. The second half of the book is devoted to in vivo protocols commonly used to evaluate the innate immune response in the mouse, including mouse models of respiratory infection, gastrointestinal inflammation, fungal and parasitic diseases, sepsis, and HIV-1 infection. It is my sincere hope that *Mouse Models of Innate Immunity* will serve the research community by providing expert advice and protocols that allow both experienced and novice investigators to successfully plan, implement, and assess disease processes associated with the innate immune response.

Blacksburg, VA, USA ***Irving C. Allen***

Contents

Contributors

IRVING C. ALLEN • *Department of Biomedical Sciences and Pathobiology, Virginia-Maryland Regional College of Veterinary Medicine, Virginia Polytechnic Institute and State University, Blacksburg, VA, USA*

BRIANNE R. BARKER • *Biology Department, Drew University, Madison, NJ, USA*

BRADFORD K. BERGES • *Department of Microbiology and Molecular Biology, Brigham Young University, Provo, UT, USA*

KEVIN R. BRAUGHTON • *Laboratory of Human Bacterial Pathogenesis, Rocky Mountain Laboratories, National Institute of Allergy and Infectious Diseases, National Institutes of Health, Hamilton, MT, USA*

THOMAS C. BRODNICKI • *Immunology and Diabetes, St Vincent's Institute of Medical Research, Fitzroy, VIC, Australia*

GERMAN I. CUADRA • *Department of Microbiology and Molecular Biology, Brigham Young University, Provo, UT, USA*

BECKLEY K. DAVIS • *Department of Biology, Franklin & Marshall College, Lancaster, PA, USA*

FRANK R. DELEO • *Rocky Mountain Laboratories, National Institute of Allergy and Infectious Diseases, National Institutes of Health, Hamilton, MT, USA*

CHRISTIAN ENGWERDA • *Immunology and Infection Laboratory, Queensland Institute of Medical Research, Herston, QLD, Australia*

CHARLES W. FREVERT • *Division of Pulmonary and Critical Care Medicine, Department of Comparative Medicine, University of Washington, Seattle, WA, USA*

MICHAEL GLOGAUER • *Faculties of Medicine & Dentistry, University of Toronto, Toronto, ON, Canada*

DENIS GRIS • *Division of Immunology, Department of Pediatrics, Faculty of Medicine, University of Sherbrooke, Sherbrooke, QC, Canada*

ASHRAFUL HAQUE • *Malaria Immunology Laboratory, Queensland Institute of Medical Research, Herston, QLD, Australia*

MARK HEISE • *Department of Genetics, The University of North Carolina, Chapel Hill, NC, USA*

EMILIE IMBEAULT • *Department of Biochemistry, Faculty of Medicine, University of Sherbrooke, Sherbrooke, QC, Canada*

BRIAN JOHNSON • *Division of Pulmonary and Critical Care Medicine, Department of Comparative Medicine, University of Washington, Seattle, WA, USA*

SCOTT D. KOBAYASHI • *Laboratory of Human Bacterial Pathogenesis, Rocky Mountain Laboratories, National Institute of Allergy and Infectious Diseases, National Institutes of Health, Hamilton, MT, USA*

YU LEI • *Department of Diagnostic Sciences, School of Dental Medicine, University of Pittsburgh Medical Center, Pittsburgh, PA, USA*

KRISTIN M. LONG • *Department of Genetics, The University of North Carolina, Chapel Hill, NC, USA*
DONNA M. MACCALLUM • *Aberdeen Fungal Group, Institute of Medical Sciences, University of Aberdeen, Aberdeen, UK*
NATALIA MALACHOWA • *Laboratory of Human Bacterial Pathogenesis, Rocky Mountain Laboratories, National Institute of Allergy and Infectious Diseases, National Institutes of Health, Hamilton, MT, USA*
CHRIS B. MOORE • *Antiviral Discovery, GlaxoSmithKline, Research Triangle Park, Durham, NC, USA*
MARCELA MONTES DE OCA • *Immunology and Infection Laboratory, Queensland Institute of Medical Research, Herston, QLD, Australia*
STANTON J. NIELSEN • *Department of Microbiology and Molecular Biology, Brigham Young University, Provo, UT, USA*
KOTA V. RAMANA • *Department of Biochemistry and Molecular Biology, University of Texas Medical Branch, Galveston, TX, USA*
KELLY RONEY • *RTI International, Research Triangle Park, Durham, NC, USA*
FREDDY M. SANCHEZ • *Department of Microbiology and Molecular Biology, Brigham Young University, Provo, UT, USA*
CATHERINE J. SANDERS • *Department of Immunology, St. Jude Children's Research Hospital, Memphis, TN, USA*
MONIKA SCHNEIDER • *Infectious and Inflammatory Disease Center, Sanford Burnham Medical Research Institute, La Jolla, CA, USA*
PHILIP M. SHERMAN • *Faculties of Medicine & Dentistry, University of Toronto, Toronto, ON, Canada*
RICHARD A. STRUGNELL • *Microbiology and Immunology, The University of Melbourne, Parkville, VIC, Australia*
XIAOLUN SUN • *Center for Gastrointestinal Biology and Disease, University of North Carolina at Chapel Hill, Chapel Hill, NC, USA*
YUE SUN • *Lineberger Comprehensive Cancer Center, University of North Carolina at Chapel Hill, Chapel Hill, NC, USA*
ANNE TANNER • *Department of Microbiology and Molecular Biology, Brigham Young University, Provo, UT, USA*
PAUL G. THOMAS • *Department of Immunology, St. Jude Children's Research Hospital, Memphis, TN, USA*
JOSHUA URONIS • *Institute for Genome Sciences and Policy, Duke University, Durham, NC, USA*
LINDA VONG • *Faculty of Medicine, University of Toronto, Toronto, ON, Canada*
NANCY WANG • *Immunology and Diabetes, St Vincent's Institute of Medical Research, Fitzroy, VIC, Australia*
HAITAO WEN • *Lineberger Comprehensive Cancer Center, The University of North Carolina at Chapel Hill, Chapel Hill, NC, USA*
DOUGLAS G. WIDMAN • *Department of Epidemiology, The University of North Carolina at Chapel Hill, Chapel Hill, NC, USA*

ODILIA L. WIJBURG • *Microbiology and Immunology, The University of Melbourne, Parkville, VIC, Australia*
UMESH C.S. YADAV • *Department of Biochemistry and Molecular Biology, University of Texas Medical Branch, Galveston, TX, USA*
ALBERT G. ZIMMERMANN • *Lineberger Comprehensive Cancer Center, University of North Carolina at Chapel Hill, Chapel Hill, NC, USA*

Chapter 1

Conventional Murine Gene Targeting

Albert G. Zimmermann and Yue Sun

Abstract

Murine gene knockout models engineered over the last two decades have continued to demonstrate their potential as invaluable tools in understanding the role of gene function in the context of normal human development and disease. The more recent elucidation of the human and mouse genomes through sequencing has opened up the capability to elucidate the function of every human gene. State-of-the-art mouse model generation allows, through a multitude of experimental steps requiring careful standardization, gene function to be reliably and predictably ablated in a live model system. The application of these standardized methodologies to directly target gene function through murine gene knockout has to date provided comprehensive and verifiable genetic models that have contributed tremendously to our understanding of the cellular and molecular pathways underlying normal and disease states in humans. The ensuing chapter provides an overview of the latest steps and procedures required to ablate gene function in a murine model.

Key words Murine gene knockout, Embryonic stem cells, Gene-targeting vector, Homologous recombination, Embryonic stem cell electroporation, Embryonic stem cell screening, Blastocyst isolation, Microinjection, Blastocyst implantation, Chimeric mice, Germline transmission

1 Introduction

Humans share between 70 and 90 % genetic similarity with mice [1]. This genetic homology results in extensive biochemical, physiological, and anatomical conservation between species and has contributed to the rise of mice as the principal animal model in the life sciences. Examples of research fields in which knockout mice have been extensively employed include cancer, hypertension, arteriosclerosis, neurological disorders, and immune-related diseases. In addition, knockout mice are currently becoming more prominently featured in the biological and scientific context of devising novel therapeutics, pharmacologics, and diagnostics. The unique benefit of mouse models is that they can, unlike human subjects, be designed to have both a defined genotype and a congenic relative to serve as an experimental control. The prior assemblage of several scientific and

Irving C. Allen (ed.), *Mouse Models of Innate Immunity: Methods and Protocols*, Methods in Molecular Biology, vol. 1031, DOI 10.1007/978-1-62703-481-4_1, © Springer Science+Business Media, LLC 2013

technological breakthroughs including the manipulation of large genomic DNA fragments, the identification and isolation of embryonic stem cells, the process of homologous recombination, and the development of methods for in vitro embryo manipulation and implantation underlies our current ability to generate genetically modified mouse models [2–4]. In addition, the establishment of institutional core facilities and private enterprises geared toward the production and support of genetically engineered mouse models have led to further explosive growth in their use.

Conceptually, the production of mice with a targeted mutation is sequentially dependent on the following critical steps: (1) identify the gene to be modified and acquire the corresponding genomic DNA sequence; (2) generate a plasmid, known as a gene-targeting vector, that includes genomic DNA sequence with the knockout mutation of interest; (3) introduce the mutation into embryonic stem (ES) cells by transferring the plasmid into these cells such that the altered sequence in the targeting vector is able to undergo homologous recombination with the endogenous genomic DNA, thereby introducing the desired modification into the ES cell genome; (4) inject the genetically modified ES cells into blastocyst-stage mouse embryos with the goal to successfully integrate the ES cells with the blastocyst inner cell mass; (5) generate viable embryos through proper implantation resulting in F0-generation chimeric mice; (6) identify germline transmission of the desired trait by breeding, which results in N1-generation animals that are heterozygous for the mutation of interest; and (7) interbreed N1-generation mice in order to produce animals that are homozygous for the intended genetic deletion.

In this chapter, we summarize current techniques involved in the generation of a gene-targeted mouse model engineered to ablate the expression of a specific endogenous mouse gene, also known as a knockout mouse. Additional technical details for each step can be gleaned from a multitude of previously published scientific articles, reviews, and manuals [2–9].

2 Materials

2.1 Gene-Targeting Vector

1. Targeting vector plasmid DNA.
2. BAC clone containing the gene of interest or C57BL/6 genomic DNA.
3. Polymerase chain reaction reagents, materials, and a thermal cycler.
4. Restriction cloning reagents (restriction enzymes, T4 DNA ligase) or recombination cloning kit.
5. DNA miniprep and PCR purification kit.
6. DH5α competent bacterial cells.

7. Gel electrophoresis apparatus and reagents (agarose, ethidium bromide, DNA molecular weight markers).
8. QIAfilter Plasmid Maxi Kit (QIAGEN).
9. Small-volume spectrophotometer.

2.2 Embryonal Stem Cell Electroporation and Selection

1. C57BL/6N-PRX-B6N #1 ES cells (Jackson Laboratory) and MEFs (C57BL/6J, Jackson Laboratory).
2. Targeting DNA construct.
3. Automated cell counter.
4. BioRad Gene Pulser electroporation system and cuvettes.
5. Tissue culture incubator: Humidified, 37 °C, 5 % CO_2.
6. Tissue culture hood.
7. Inverted microscope.
8. ES cell medium: 82 % DMEM (high glucose), 15 % FBS (heat inactivated), 100 μM β-mercaptoethanol, 2 mM L-glutamine, 0.1 mM MEM non-essential amino acids, 1 mM sodium pyruvate, penicillin (50–100 U/ml), streptomycin (50–100 μg/ml), 1,000 U/ml leukemia inhibitory factor.
9. Trypsin–EDTA.
10. Geneticin (G418), ganciclovir (9-(1, 3-dihydroxy-2-propoxymethyl) guanine), and mitomycin C.
11. Dulbecco's PBS.
12. Gelatinized tissue culture plates coated with MEF feeder cells.

2.3 Embryonal Stem Cell Screening

1. TaKaRa LA Taq with 10× PCR buffer and dNTP mixture.
2. PCR primers.
3. Southern blot reagents (Digoxigenin system; Roche).

2.4 Mouse Blastocyst Isolation

1. C57BL/6/BrdCrHsd-*Tyr*^{c} (Harlan Laboratories) or B6(Cg)-*Tyr*$^{c\text{-}2J}$/J (Jackson Laboratory) albino male and female breeders.
2. Pregnant mare serum (PMS) and human chorionic gonadotropin (hCG).
3. Mouth-controlled aspirator tube assembly for microcapillary pipettes (Sigma-Aldrich).
4. Dissecting microscope with illuminator.
5. Dissecting instruments (fine-pointed scissors, regular and fine straight and curved forceps).
6. Syringes (10 ml) and needles (25 G).
7. Micropipette puller (Sutter Instruments) and glass capillary tubes (1 mm).
8. EmbryoMax M2 and KSOM medium (Millipore).
9. Embryo-tested mineral oil (Sigma-Aldrich).

2.5 ES Cell Preparation

1. Gelatinized tissue culture plates coated with MEF feeder cells.

2.6 Blastocyst Microinjection

1. Inverted microscope with mechanical stage and movable objectives.
2. Hydraulic manual micromanipulator (Eppendorf CellTram Oil) and microinjector (Eppendorf Celltram Vario).

2.7 Preparation of Pseudo-Pregnant Recipient Mice

1. Female CD-1 mice (Charles River).
2. Male CD-1 mice (Charles River), vasectomized.

2.8 Embryo Transfer to Recipient Female Mice

1. Pseudo-pregnant female CD-1 mice, 2.5 dpc.
2. Avertin (2, 2, 2,-Tribromoethanol).
3. Surgical instruments (fine-pointed scissors, regular and fine straight and curved forceps, endoscopic vascular bulldog clamp).
4. Surgical suture (Ethicon).
5. Autoclip wound closing system (BD Diagnostic Systems).
6. Small heating pad.

2.9 Germline Transmission

1. Mouse housing and husbandry facility with veterinary care, approved by the Association for Assessment and Accreditation of Laboratory Animal Care International (AAALAC).
2. Institutional Animal Care and Use Committee (IACUC)-approved Animal Protocol.
3. Mouse identification system (ear notch or ear tag).
4. Tail clip genotyping protocol.

3 Methods

3.1 Gene-Targeting Vector

1. Identify the gene to be targeted and isolate the region of interest from the mouse genome. Most commonly, mouse genomic regions encompassing genes or gene segments can be obtained from bacterial artificial chromosomes (BAC) clones (UCSC Genome Browser, genome.ucsc.edu). If a BAC clone is not available, suitable DNA fragments for targeting vector construction can be generated through a PCR-based cloning approach. To ablate function, it is critical to target a region of the gene that is critical for normal activity. Gene expression can be affected by targeting transcriptional regulatory sequences through the disruption of promoter function or more commonly by disrupting critical exons at the proximal end of the gene. The disruption of normal protein expression and function is thus achieved by replacing regulatory sequences or an exon deemed critical for

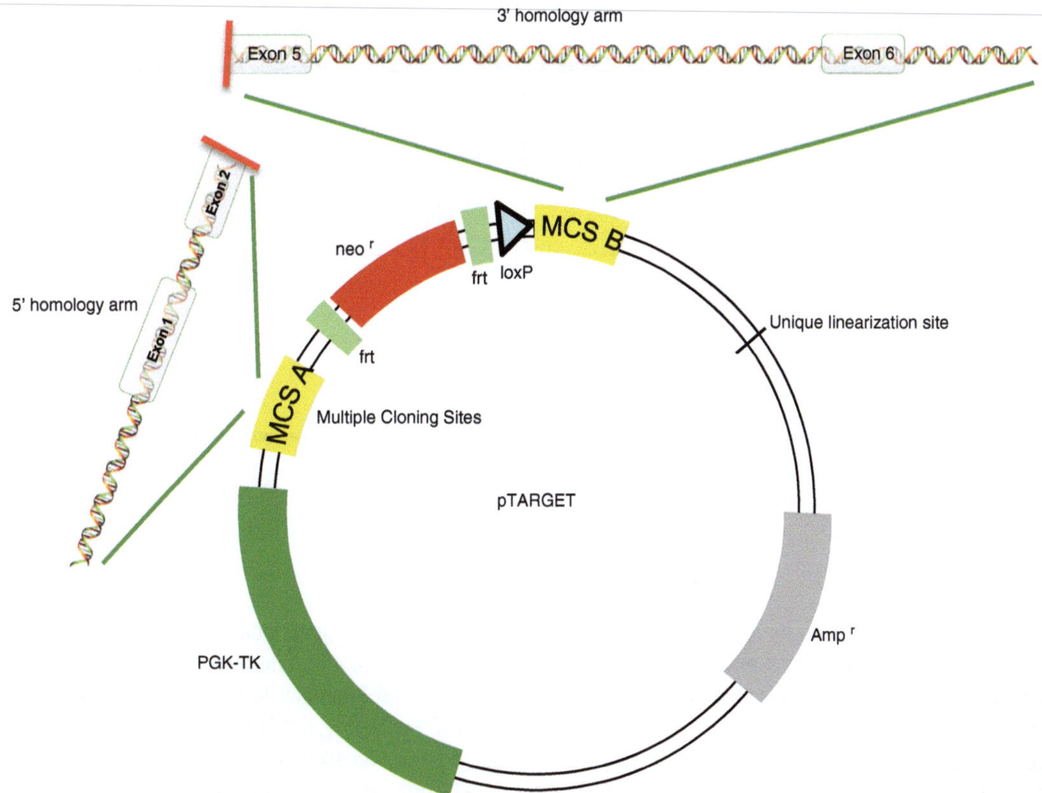

Fig. 1 Prototypical gene targeting vector with 5′ and 3′ homology arms and a positive and negative selection cassette. A targeting vector containing two arms of homology is designed to excise Exons 3 and 4 from a prospective 12-exon gene. The vector contains the neomycin antibiotic resistance gene cassette (neo^r) for positive selection, conferring resistance to geneticin (G418). In addition, the vector contains a PGK-TK gene, the product of which is capable of converting ganciclovir into toxic metabolic intermediaries, for negative selection. Cells that undergo homologous recombination will be geneticin and ganciclovir resistant. Cells that contain a randomly integrated targeting vector will likely retain both the neo^r and PGK-TK genes and, although geneticin resistant, will be ganciclovir sensitive

function with a positive selection cassette that expresses the bacterial antibiotic resistance gene neomycin (neo^r) (Fig. 1) (*see* **Note 1**). In addition to ablating gene function, the neomycin cassette confers resistance to the antibiotic geneticin, which will also permit for the selection of ES cells that contain the desired genetic modification. To precisely target the gene of interest, the targeting vector will need to encompass two arms of homology that contain DNA sequences that are identical to the genomic sequence directly adjacent to the region to be "knocked out," and being replaced by the neo^r cassette. Furthermore, to optimize homologous recombination it is important that the targeting vector arms of homology consist of DNA that is genetically isogenic to the mouse strain to be targeted. To prevent nonhomologous or random integration

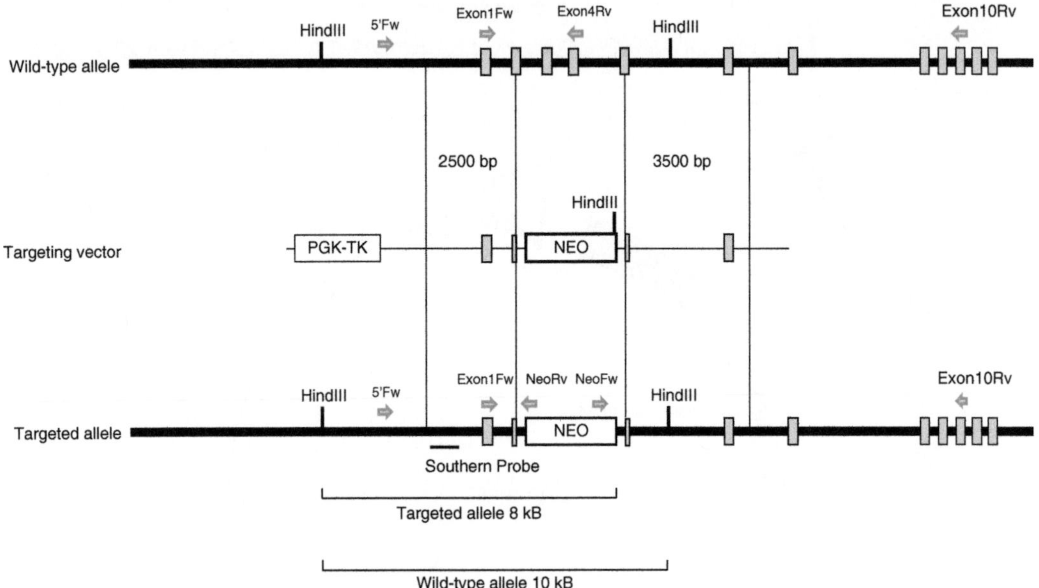

Fig. 2 Targeting approach for ablating the gene function of a hypothetical gene locus by homologous recombination. Diagrammatic representation of the PCR strategy employed to confirm homologous recombination in ES cells using a combination of primers located both externally and internally to the DNA sequence being replaced as well as covering both 5′ and 3′ arms of homology (5′Fw/NeoRv, NeoFw/Exon10Rv). Southern blot analysis using the restriction enzyme site *HindIII* and a labeled probe will allow for the differentiation between the wild-type, 10 kb allele and the targeted, 8 kb allele. Finally, primers internal to the region of homologous recombination can be used for genotyping purposes once the animal model has been established (Exon1Fw/Exon4Rv/NeoRv)

of the targeting vector, in addition to positive selection (neo^r), a second negative selection step is employed that utilizes the herpes simplex virus-thymidine kinase (TK) gene driven by the phosphoglycerate kinase (PGK) promoter (PGK-TK). The viral TK protein will convert the substrate precursor ganciclovir, a guanine analogue, to a toxic metabolite that interferes with cellular DNA synthesis and ultimately results in cell death. The PGK-TK selection cassette is placed outside of the region of homologous recombination, and thus will select against ES cells in which nonhomologous or random integration events have occurred (Figs. 1 and 2).

2. The availability of a BAC clone for the gene of interest will dictate the approach taken to generate the targeting vector. In the absence of a suitable contiguous BAC clone, a genomic PCR and restriction enzyme cloning approach will have to be utilized to generate a properly engineered targeting vector. Targeting vector design and construction are typically executed by academic core facilities and commercial enterprises, but generic gene-targeting vector backbones can still be obtained for custom vector engineering (examples include Thermo Scientific, OSDupDel Vectors).

3. Several basic requirements need to be met to successfully design a targeting vector. The targeting vector needs to contain two arms of homology, each of which should be between 2 and 5 kb in length. When utilizing a PCR-based approach, two homology arms are generated and cloned upstream and downstream of the neo^r-positive selection cassette into a vector containing a preexisting negative selection cassette (PGK-TK) and an ampicillin resistance gene for bacterial DNA amplification (Amp^r) (Fig. 1). Alternatively, the targeting vector can be generated and customized through the use of recombineering methodologies, which obviate the need for cumbersome cloning strategies [10]. The latter approach allows for the subcloning of the genomic target sequence obtained from a BAC clone directly into an appropriate targeting vector. Stepwise, other components, e.g., a neo^r-positive selection cassette and restriction sites for future Southern blot analysis, can be engineered into desired locations of the targeting sequence.
4. Amplify the targeting vector plasmid DNA for ES cell electroporation. To accomplish this, the plasmid DNA will need to be transformed into competent *Escherichia coli* bacterial cells (most commonly DH5α) according to the manufacturer's protocol for competent cells and then amplified/purified according to the manufacturer's instructions for the QIAfilter Plasmid Maxi DNA affinity purification kit.
5. Linearize the resulting plasmid DNA at a unique restriction site. Targeting vector linearization facilitates the process of homologous recombination upon ES cell electroporation (*see* **Note 2**). In order to provide sufficient plasmid DNA (40 μg of DNA is required for two independent transfections), linearize 100 μg of the targeting vector using the restriction enzyme specific for the unique linearization site, according to the manufacturer's instructions (Fig. 1). Following restriction digestion, verify, through gel electrophoresis (analyze 200 ng of DNA), that the targeting vector was digested to completion. Quantitate the DNA by small-volume spectrophotometry and store for future electroporation into mouse ES cells.

3.2 Embryonic Stem Cell Electroporation and Selection

1. Choose an ES cell line for gene targeting. Several ES cell lines are available; however, one of the most commonly used models for genetically modified mouse studies is the murine line C57BL/6. This line is a standardized and widely referenced inbred laboratory mouse strain used in comparative animal studies. Furthermore, the genomic sequence of the C57BL/6 mouse strain has been determined [1, 11]. In addition, several groups have succeeded in generating culture- and implantation-competent ES cell lines from this strain [12, 13], which are now commercially available for gene targeting

(C57BL/6N-PRX-B6N #1) (*see* **Note 3**). In addition, C57BL/6 blastocysts were found to be efficient hosts for the implantation of these co-isogenic ES cells [14] resulting in the establishment of embryo donor lines that can be easily obtained from Harlan Laboratories (C57BL/6/BrdCrHsd-*Tyr*^{c}) and Jackson Laboratory (B6(Cg)-*Tyr*$^{c\text{-}2J}$/J). Coat color screening, similar to the previously used coat-color determining gene agouti, can now also be realized by using the above-listed albino C57BL/6 strain blastocysts that are isogenic to the "black" C57BL/6 ES cells employed for electroporation (C57BL/6N-PRX-B6N #1). C57BL/6 mice with the albino phenotype contain a spontaneous recessive point mutation in the tyrosinase gene (*Tyr*^{c}). Blastocysts obtained from these animals have been found to be more efficacious than other albino lines in generating chimeric, germline-competent mice [14, 15]. Electroporation continues to be the method of choice to introduce targeting vector DNA into ES cells since it is reliable and reproducible.

2. On the day of electroporation, trypsinize two to four 100 mm plates containing 50–80 % confluent ES cells. Neutralize the trypsin using ES cell medium and wash the cells twice in D-PBS. Electroporate 1×10^7 cells in the presence of 20 μg of DNA using a Bio-Rad Gene Pulser set at 250 V and 500 μF.
3. Following transfection the ES cells are plated onto twelve 100 mm plates containing a feeder layer of mouse embryo fibroblasts (MEFs) that have been cultured on a gelatinized substrate and cell cycle arrested using mitomycin C [16, 17]. MEFs are required to support the growth of the electroporated ES cells and to prevent premature differentiation.
4. Twenty-four hours post transfection, place the ES cells under selection using G418 (150–400 μg/ml) and ganciclovir (1 μM). Resistant ES cells will grow clonally within 8–12 days to aggregates of macroscopic size.
5. Using a pipet tip, transfer single clones from up to 192 colonies to a 96-well plate (up to 2 plates). Dissociate the cell aggregates using trypsin–EDTA and transfer 50 % of the sample to a 96-well PCR plate. In parallel, a "master plate" suitable for tissue culture expansion needs to be frozen down (using the remaining 50 % of cells) for future manipulation of positive clones.
6. Genomic DNA from the individual ES cell clones present in the 96-well PCR plate is generated by the addition of 12.5 μl of 25 mM NaOH/0.2 mM EDTA. The plate is incubated at 95 °C for 60 min. The alkaline hydrolysis reaction is terminated by the addition of 12.5 μl of 40 mM Tris–HCl. One microliter of the resulting lysate is used for high-throughput PCR screening.

3.3 Embryonal Stem Cell Screening

1. Identify ES cell clones that have undergone correct homologous recombination. The electroporated targeting construct will undergo a unique low-frequency (1–5 %) event called homologous recombination. Homologous recombination is a genetic occurrence in which nucleotide sequences are exchanged between two very similar or identical regions of DNA. The previously described arms of homology included in the targeting vector will facilitate the exchange of identical DNA sequences and thus result in the introduction of the neo^r selection marker into the gene to be targeted. Due to the fact that most genes are represented by two copies or alleles, only one isoform of the targeted gene will be affected. Exceptions include genes that are located on the X or Y chromosome and are subsequently to be studied in male animals. The functional importance of X and Y chromosome-linked genes can be more cumbersome to study since modification of a single active allele might result in embryonic lethality, thereby limiting the ability of chimeric male mice to generate subsequent generations of offspring. To identify ES cell clones that have undergone correct homologous recombination, colonies will be screened for the proper targeting of the allele of interest. Commonly, the primary screening method will be PCR based due to the high-throughput characteristics of this approach (Fig. 3a). PCR-positive clones will be confirmed using the technique of Southern blotting, which relies on the identification of the correctly targeted allele based on the presence of a unique restriction enzyme site within the targeted sequence versus the wild-type genomic locus (Fig. 2). Restriction digestion of the genomic DNA is followed by size resolution using gel electrophoresis, membrane blotting, and binding to a specific DNA probe (Fig. 3b). Finally, a multiplex genotyping PCR protocol (for example Exon1Fw/Exon4Rv/NeoRv) will need to be devised to allow for the straightforward detection of and discrimination between the wild-type and targeted allele in the final animal model (Figs. 2 and 3c) (*see* **Note 4**).
2. Utilize long-range PCR to evaluate integration. Since partial homologous recombination can occur, it is important to screen both the upstream and downstream homology arms of the targeted allele for proper integration. The most effective approach is to design a methodology combining primers (5'Fw/NeoRv and NeoFw/Exon10Rv) located within and outside of the region of homologous recombination and that covers both proximal and distal regions of the targeting arms (Figs. 2 and 3a). Robust PCR screening results can be realized with the TaKaRa LA Taq polymerase used according to the manufacturer's protocol.

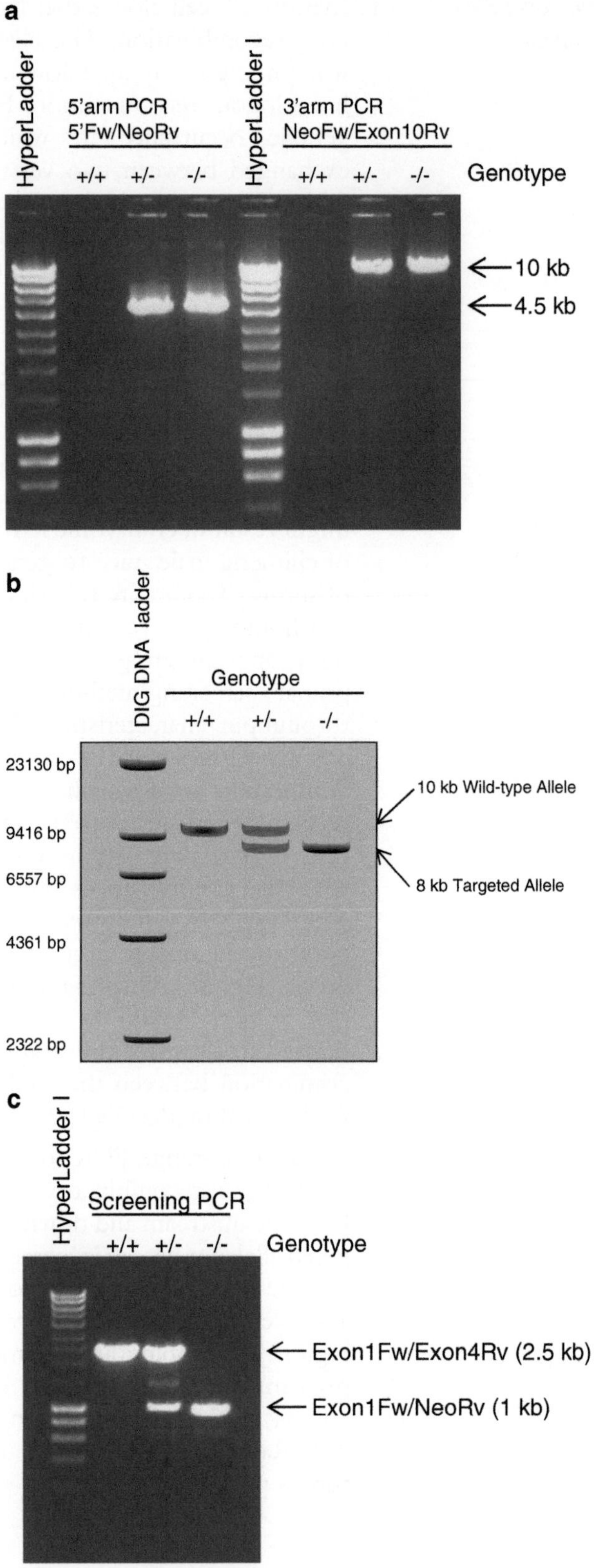

a
HyperLadder I
5'arm PCR
5'Fw/NeoRv
HyperLadder I
3'arm PCR
NeoFw/Exon10Rv
+/+ +/- -/-
+/+ +/- -/-
Genotype
10 kb
4.5 kb
b
DIG DNA ladder
Genotype
+/+ +/- -/-
23130 bp
9416 bp
6557 bp
4361 bp
2322 bp
10 kb Wild-type Allele
8 kb Targeted Allele
c
HyperLadder I
Screening PCR
+/+ +/- -/-
Genotype
Exon1Fw/Exon4Rv (2.5 kb)
Exon1Fw/NeoRv (1 kb)

3. Upon identification of PCR-positive clones, expand the selected ES cell colonies from the master plate onto 24-well plates. This will generate a large amount of cells from each positive clone for subsequent genomic DNA isolation, a necessary requirement for PCR reconfirmation and Southern blot analysis. In addition, each positive clone will be frozen for liquid nitrogen storage and future ES cell expansion for blastocyst microinjection (*see* Protocol 3.6) [17].

4. Perform Southern blot analysis employing a restriction site outside of, and a unique site within, the region of homologous recombination (in this case HindIII) to confirm correct homologous integration (Figs. 2 and 3b). Southern blotting allows for accurate size assessment of the gene-targeted allele compared to the unmodified allelic DNA (8 kb versus 10 kb) and will also assist in the detection of alternate copies of non-homologously integrated targeting vector DNA (Fig. 3b). The Roche Digoxigenin system provides an all-encompassing approach to Southern blot analysis.

3.4 Mouse Blastocyst Isolation

1. To generate sufficient embryos for microinjection 10 female mice are induced to superovulate. To initiate superovulation, each female mouse receives an intraperitoneal (IP) injection containing five international units (IU) of PMS at noon followed by an IP injection of 5 IU of hCG after 46–48 h. Immediately following the hCG injection the female animals are mated with male mice. Mice that exhibit a vaginal plug the next morning are considered 0.5 days post coitus (dpc) and are isolated from their male counterparts and caged separately for 3 days (e.g., administer PMS on Thursday, followed by hCG on Saturday, immediately set up matings, separate plugged females on Sunday, collect embryos on Wednesday morning). Resulting blastocyst embryos are subsequently isolated and prepared for microinjection [5, 6]. The blastocyst yield from

Fig. 3 (continued) Screening protocol to identify gene-targeted mice using a PCR-based approach as well as Southern blot analysis. (**a**) The external PCR primers (5′Fw and Exon10Rv) in conjunction with the internal primers (NeoRV and NeoFw) are used on genomic DNA (ear notch or tail clip biopsy) to verify correct targeting. Only following homologous recombination are the two primer sets juxtaposed and able to generate 4.5 and 10 kb PCR products, respectively. (**b**) Genomic DNA from a gene-targeted mouse is subjected to Southern blot analysis to verify correct targeting. (**c**) Once the animal model has been established genomic DNA will act as a template for the multiplex genotyping PCR primer pairs Exon1Fw/Exon4Rv and Exon1Fw/NeoRv to amplify a specific 2.5 kb PCR product for the wild-type allele and a shorter 1 kb product for the gene-targeted allele as evidenced by size separation employing agarose gel electrophoresis

10 superovulated mice can vary from 60 to 100 embryos or more, 80 % of which will generally be at the optimal developmental stage for ES cell injection.

2. Humanely euthanize female donor mice at 3.5 dpc using CO_2 asphyxiation/cervical dislocation.
3. Place the animal with the ventral side facing up. Surgically remove the uterus after making incisions in the abdominal wall to expose the reproductive tract.
4. Excise the uterus by gripping the cervix with forceps and cutting through the vaginal tissue.
5. Place the collected uteri in a 6 cm dish containing EmbryoMax M2 medium and detach the uterine horns from the cervix.
6. Under a dissecting microscope, employing a 25 G needle attached to a 10 ml syringe containing M2 medium, flush the fertilized blastocysts from each uterine horn with approximately 0.5 ml of medium.
7. Collect the embryos with a mouth-controlled aspirator tube assembly with an attached capillary pipette and place in a droplet of medium under embryo-tested mineral oil for the same-day ES cell microinjection. Properly aged and matured embryos will exhibit a clearly visible blastocoel cavity and a surrounding intact zona pellucida. Embryos that, at the time of harvest, are not fully developed can be incubated in EmbryoMax KSOM medium for several hours at 37 °C to allow for blastocoel formation.

3.5 ES Cell Preparation

1. On the day of blastocyst injection, targeted ES cells from a 60–70 % confluent 6 cm dish are trypsinized, washed with medium, and suspended in 1 ml of ES cell medium [17]. A small volume containing ES cells is transferred to a droplet of medium adjacent to the one containing the blastocysts awaiting microinjection [6].

3.6 Blastocyst Microinjection

1. Microinjection of the blastocyst is performed on the lid of a 6 cm petri dish in a large droplet of ES cell medium submerged under embryo-tested mineral oil [5, 6].
2. A single embryo is immobilized by slight negative pressure using a holding capillary attached to a CellTram Oil. The inner cell mass should be oriented toward the opening of the holding capillary.
3. Employing a glass transfer capillary attached to a CellTram Vario, approach the blastocyst from the opposite side, puncture the zona pellucida between the trophectoderm cells, and expel between 10 and 15 ES cells that are lined up single file into the blastocoel cavity using slight positive pressure.

4. Generally, a total of 14–16 injected blastocysts are needed for successful implantation into a pseudo-pregnant female (*see* Protocol 3.8) recipient that is 8–10 weeks or older. Commonly, two independently isolated and targeted ES cell lines will be injected into blastocysts on separate days to improve the probability of obtaining chimeric offspring.

3.7 Preparation of Pseudo-Pregnant Recipient Mice

1. The generation of viable offspring from the injected blastocysts requires the implantation into recipient female mice. The CD-1 line is one of several commercially available foster lines that are used as recipient mice due to their vigorous reproductive performance and nonaggressive behavior. Mating of recipient female mice with male mice is necessary to establish the hormonal conditions favoring the implantation and normal development of the manipulated embryos. Since the recipient female mice should not be fertilized, they are mated with vasectomized males [5].
2. To prime the uterus to accept and maintain transferred embryos the recipient female mice need to be physiologically synchronized with the developmental stage of the implanted embryos. Thus, female foster mice are mated 2.5 days prior to embryo implantation (e.g., set up matings on Sunday, check for plugs on Monday morning, separate animals, implant embryos on Wednesday).
3. The timing of recipient mating is established visually by the presence of a mating plug in female mice at day 0.5 post coitus. At this time the recipient mice are separated from their male partners and kept until embryo implantation.
4. In order to generate sufficient pseudo-pregnant female mice for embryo implantation approximately 35 mating pairs are arranged for each embryo transfer day, generally resulting in approximately 6–12 reproductively primed foster females [5, 6].

3.8 Embryo Transfer to Recipient Female Mice

1. Manipulated blastocysts are implanted into recipient females as soon as possible after completion of the ES cell microinjection. Approximately 14–16 embryos are implanted into the uterine horns of a pseudo-pregnant CD-1 recipient female mouse mated 2.5 days previously with a vasectomized male.
2. The recipient female mouse is anesthetized by an IP injection of 0.2 ml/10 g body weight of 2.5 % Avertin.
3. The animal is placed on its ventral side and hair removed from an area on the right and left side of the back, two-thirds down from the head.
4. Employing aseptic surgical technique, a small 1 cm dorsal incision (rostrocaudal axis) is made, approximately midway dorsoventral, that reaches through both the skin and peritoneum. The uterus should be directly underneath the incision.

5. Place the animal under a dissecting microscope and expose the uterus by grabbing the fat pad surrounding the reproductive organ and slowly and carefully pulling the ovary, oviduct, and uterus through the incision.
6. Secure the fat pad with an endoscopic vascular bulldog clamp that is positioned to the opposite side of the mouse's back to prevent the uterus from retracting into the body cavity.
7. Carefully collect the blastocysts with a mouth-controlled aspirator tube assembly attached to a capillary transfer pipette.
8. Stabilize the uterus with a pair of fine forceps and carefully transfer the blastocysts into the uterine horn by piercing the uterine wall and slowly, with the use of positive pressure, injecting the embryos into the uterine cavity.
9. Retract the capillary pipette and remove the bulldog clamp. Gently push the reproductive organs back into the peritoneal cavity. Close the peritoneal incision with surgical suture and staple the skin with a surgical wound clip.
10. Let the animals recover on a warm heating pad until they regain consciousness. Return the mice to the animal housing facility and monitor for 24 hours for potential complications.
11. The pups resulting from manipulated embryos will be born around 18 days post transfer [5].
12. Successfully implanted embryos will result in offspring exhibiting an agouti-like coat color appearance, approximately 2 weeks after birth when coat color becomes apparent. This chimeric coat color is the result of the contribution of the injected "black" C57BL/6 ES cells to the "white" albino (C57BL/6/BrdCrHsd-*Tyr*^{c}, B6(Cg)-*Tyr*$^{c\text{-}2J}$/J) blastocyst background (Figs. 4 and 5a). Pups can generally be weaned at 21 days of age [5, 6].

3.9 Germline Transmission

1. The most critical step in the development of a gene knockout mouse model is the generation of the ES–embryo chimera that will transmit the genetic modification to subsequent generations. The recent establishment of albino C57BL/6 embryo donor strains (C57BL/6/BrdCrHsd-*Tyr*^{c}, C57BL/6(Cg)-*Tyr*$^{c\text{-}2J}$/J) has made the generation of a gene-targeted C57BL/6 isogenic line incredibly easy [18]. In addition, albino C57BL/6 blastocyst hosts obviate the previously required and time-consuming nine-generation backcrossing scheme into the C57BL/6 line necessary when using the historically employed B6D2F1/J donor strain (F1 hybrid from a C57BL/6J female and DBA/2J male). When C57BL/6-derived ES cells are injected into albino C57BL/6 blastocysts, chimeric mice are generated that are phenotypically identifiable by their coat color which will consist of a mix of black fur on a white fur background (Fig. 4). The degree of chimerism can range from

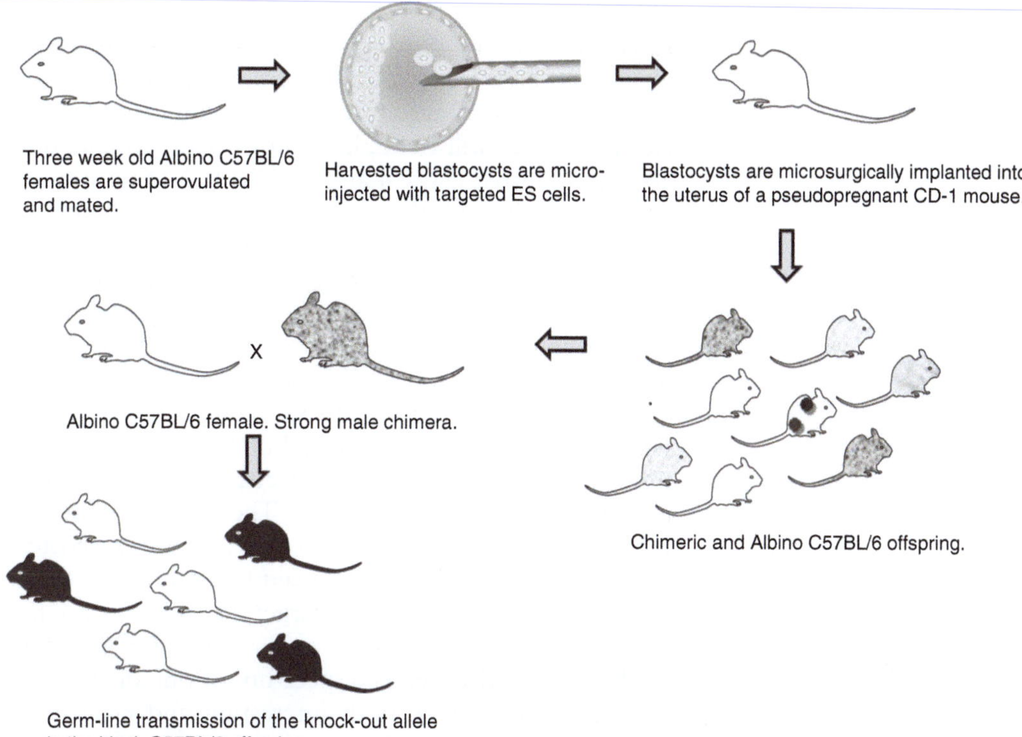

Fig. 4 Generation of knockout mice heterozygous for the targeted allele. Blastocysts obtained from albino C57BL/6 females are injected with gene-targeted C57BL/6 ES cells (10–15 cells). Fourteen to sixteen injected blastocysts are implanted into a pseudo-pregnant CD-1 recipient mouse resulting in albino and chimeric offspring, as evidenced by the degree of black coat color penetration. Highly chimeric male founders are crossed with albino C57BL/6 female mice. Germline transmission is achieved with the birth of *black pups* which will have inherited the targeted allele

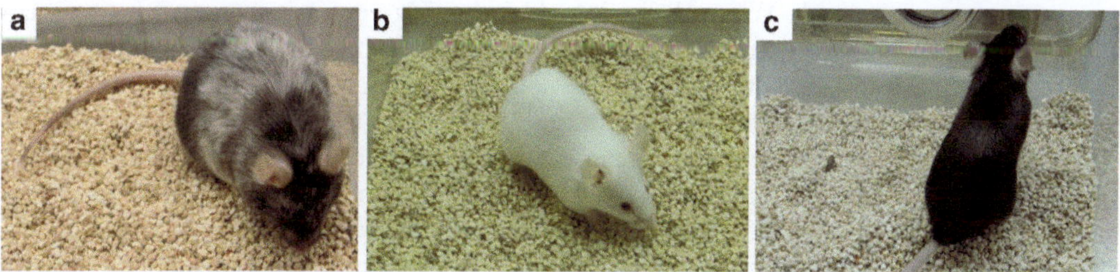

Fig. 5 Mice employed for model generation. A transmitting male chimeric mouse (**a**) created using gene-targeted C57BL/6-derived ES cells injected into an albino C57BL/6 blastocyst. Following breeding with an albino C57BL/6 female mouse, both albino C57BL/6(*Tyr*$^{c\text{-}2J}$/*Tyr*$^{c\text{-}2J}$) littermates (**b**) and black gene-targeted C57BL/6 founders will be generated (**c**)

a few black furry patches on a mostly white background to almost uniformly gray fur (Figs. 4 and 5a). The higher the degree of black to black fur penetration, thus representing the overall contribution of the injected ES cells to the whole animal including the reproductive organs, the more likely that germline transmission of the targeted allele will occur. Chimeric pups, as evidenced by coat color, can be weaned at 21 days post birth and breeding to obtain germline transmission initiated at 6–8 weeks of age. Strong male chimeras bred with female albino mice will yield black pups when germline transmission has occurred (Figs. 4 and 5). The lack of transmission will be obvious through the production of white albino progeny (Figs. 4 and 5). To fully realize the establishment of a new mouse model, the black offspring, heterozygous for the targeted allele, will need to be bred to the stage of genetic homozygosity. Depending on the nature and function of the targeted allele, this penultimate step can introduce a whole spectrum of additional complications. Outcomes can range in severity from strong effects, such as developmental interference resulting in no or nonviable offspring, to mild effects, such as the lack of an obvious phenotype in adult animals. These extreme outcomes will require extensive scientific scrutiny to elucidate (*see* **Notes 5** and **6**). Notwithstanding, as evidenced by a multitude of scientific publication, the advent of gene targeting technologies have contributed tremendously to our understanding of gene function in health and disease. The spectrum of outcomes in new model generation can be both interesting and challenging; however, with the arrival of a more recent technical development, tissue- and cell-specific conditional gene knockout, mostly all limitations of the conventional knockout approach can now be eclipsed (*see* **Note 7**) [9].

4 Notes

1. When designing the targeting vector it is important to guard against possible endogenous gene expression events such as alternative in-frame splicing which could result in the production of a truncated protein with altered activity, including dominant negative or gain of function characteristics. To guard against this possibility it is recommended that the neo cassette be placed such that it disrupts splice donor and/or splice acceptor sites on one or both of the exons adjacent to the exon being targeted for removal. If random splicing occurs under these circumstances, the resulting reading frame will be shifted and most likely result in the synthesis of an out-of-frame noncoding transcript that will contain premature translational stop codons.
2. Restriction enzyme linearization occurs outside of the targeting cassette and requires a unique restriction site to be present within the targeting vector.

3. Historically, 129 strain mice were used for gene targeting because their ES cells are easy to derive and manipulate and they retain their competency to repopulate the mouse germline. However, more recently it was determined that there is a large degree of genetic diversity among 129 substrains, thus making this line less attractive for comparative research.
4. Record keeping is of the utmost importance. In addition, it is necessary to verify that every step of the model generation has been executed flawlessly. Many gene targeting projects have become unhinged because of inadequate quality control, including flawed vector design, insufficient verification of correct homologous recombination through PCR screening and Southern blot analysis, inadequate care to assure ES cell competency and clonal nature, limited understanding of mouse breeding schemes to obtain germline transmission, and finally lack of straightforward genotyping methodologies to discriminate between wild-type and gene-targeted alleles.
5. Individuals working on a gene targeting project will need to have a detailed understanding of a broad range of techniques that will be required to bring the model to fruition, including molecular biology, genotyping, mouse husbandry, histology, and mouse development, anatomy, and physiology. In addition, skills related to the model at hand, which might include embryology, physiology, and immunology, will be required.
6. Generating a gene-targeted mouse model is very time consuming, requires a well-established animal housing and husbandry infrastructure, is subject to strict regulations regarding animal handling and treatment in the form of national and local laws (AAALAC, IACUC), and is capital intensive. These considerations have to be taken into account before initiating studies using animal models.
7. It is important to note that most animal models are conceptually derived from gene function observed in in vitro cell culture or empirically from the study of singular protein function. However, proteins have diverse functions and animal systems are exponentially more complex and adaptive, with the end result that some gene-targeting effects will be tremendously disruptive while other gene functions will remain elusive due to genetic and/or functional redundancy.

Acknowledgment

The software application ScienceSlides Suite 2011 (VisiScience) was used to generate Figs. 1 and 4.

References

1. Waterston RH, Lindblad-Toh K, Birney E et al (2002) Initial sequencing and comparative analysis of the mouse genome. Nature 420(6915):520–562
2. Thomas KR, Capecchi MR (1987) Site directed mutagenesis by gene targeting in mouse embryo-derived stem cells. Cell 51: 503–512
3. Doetschman T, Gregg RG, Maeda N, Hooper ML, Melton DW, Thompson S, Smithies O (1987) Targeted correction of a mutant HPRT gene in mouse embryonic stem cells. Nature 330:576–578
4. Koller BH, Hagemann LJ, Doetschman T, Hagaman JR, Huang S, Williams PJ, First NL, Maeda N, Smithies O (1989) Germ-line transmission of a planned alteration made in a hypoxanthine phosphoribosyltransferase gene by homologous recombination in embryonic stem cells. Proc Natl Acad Sci U S A 86(22): 8927–8931
5. Nagy A, Gertsenstein M, Vintersten K, Behringer R (2003) Manipulating the mouse embryo: a laboratory manual, 3rd edn. Cold Spring Harbor Laboratory Press, New York
6. Reid SW, Tessarollo L (2009) Isolation, microinjection and transfer of mouse blastocysts. Methods Mol Biol 530:269–285
7. Galli-Taliadors LA, Sedgwick JD, Wood SA, Körner H (1995) Gene knock-out technology: a methodological overview for the interested novice. J Immunol Methods 181: 1–15
8. Mak TW, Penninger JM, Ohashi P (2001) Knockout mice: a paradigm shift in modern immunology. Nat Rev immunol 1:11–19
9. Doyle A, McGarry MP, Lee NA, Lee JJ (2011) The construction of transgenic and gene knockout/knockin mouse models of human disease. Transgenic Res 29:1–23
10. Sharan SK, Thomason LC, Kuznetsov SG, Court DL (2009) Recombineering: a homologous recombination-based method of genetic engineering. Nat Protoc 4(2):206–223
11. Seong E, Saunders TL, Steward CL, Burmeister M (2004) To knockout in 129 or in C57BL/6: that is the question. Trends Genet 20(2):59–62
12. Ledermann B, Burki K (1991) Establishment of a germ-line competent C57BL/6 embryonic stem cell line. Exp Cell Res 197(2):254–258
13. Lemckert FA, Sedgwick JD, Körner H (1997) Gene targeting in C57BL/6 ES cells. Successful germ line transmission using recipient BALB/c blastocysts developmentally matured in vitro. Nucleic Acids Res 25(4):917–918
14. Schuster-Gossler K, Lee AW, Lerner CP, Parker HJ, Dyer VW, Scott VE, Gossler A, Conover JC (2001) Use of coisogenic host blastocysts for efficient establishment of germline chimeras with C57BL/6 J ES cell lines. Biotechniques 31(5):1022–1024, 1026
15. Griep AE, John MC, Ikeda S, Ikeda A (2011) Gene targeting in the mouse. Methods Mol Biol 770:293–312
16. Wang Z (2011) Derivation of mouse embryotic stem cell lines from blastocysts produced by fertilization and somatic cell nuclear transfer. Methods Mol Biol 770:529–549
17. Southon E, Tessarollo L (2009) Manipulating mouse embryonic stem cells. Methods Mol Biol 530:165–185
18. Luo C, Zuniga J, Edison E et al (2011) Superovulation strategies for 6 commonly used mouse strains. J Am Assoc Lab Anim Sci 50(4):471–478

Chapter 2

Production and Characterization of Humanized Rag2$^{-/-}\gamma c^{-/-}$ Mice

Freddy M. Sanchez, German I. Cuadra, Stanton J. Nielsen, Anne Tanner, and Bradford K. Berges

Abstract

Mice reconstituted with human immune cells represent a model to study the development and functionality of the human immune system. Recent improvements in humanized mice have resulted in multi-lineage hematopoiesis, prolonged human cell engraftment that is detectable in many mouse organs, and the ability to generate de novo human innate and adaptive immune responses. Here, we describe the methods used to produce and characterize humanized Rag2$^{-/-}\gamma c^{-/-}$ mice.

Key words Humanized mice, Animal disease models, Hematopoietic stem cells, Stem cell transplantation, RAG-hu mice, SCID-hu mice, BLT mice

1 Introduction

The preclinical evaluation of therapeutics for a variety of human diseases has relied mainly on the use of small animals and nonhuman primates. Despite the genetic traits conserved between some of these animals and humans, species-specific differences exist. Among these differences are the susceptibility to infection by microbial pathogens, and the host immune response to those infections. The discovery of the severe combined immunodeficiency mutation (*Prkdc*^{scid}) in mice (C.B-17 SCID mice) led to the first attempts to use these animals for the development of effective in vivo models that more accurately resemble the complexity of human biology [1]. One such development has been the "humanization" of mice.

Humanized mice are described as immunocompetent mice capable of transgenically expressing human genes, or immunodeficient mice capable of being engrafted with cells of human origin (typically hematopoietic stem cells, HSCs, or peripheral blood mononuclear cells, PBMCs). These models have provided important findings relevant to various fundamental aspects of human

Irving C. Allen (ed.), *Mouse Models of Innate Immunity: Methods and Protocols*, Methods in Molecular Biology, vol. 1031, DOI 10.1007/978-1-62703-481-4_2, © Springer Science+Business Media, LLC 2013

biology and immunology, including human hemato-lymphopoiesis, innate and adaptive immune responses, autoimmune diseases, infectious diseases, and cancer [2, 3]. The introduction of additional genetic modifications capable of overcoming the limitations (e.g., engraftment barriers) present in the earlier models of humanized mice has permitted a gradual optimization in the generation of such mouse models. Thus, in the past two decades various improved humanized mouse models have been developed [4, 5].

A more recent innovation in the humanization of mice was achieved by crossing mice homozygous for a deletion in the recombination activating gene 2 (Rag2) with mice homozygous for a deletion in the common gamma chain receptor (γc) [6, 7]. $Rag2^{-/-}\gamma c^{-/-}$ mice are incapable of producing mature T, B, and NK cells because Rag2 is required to generate B and T cell receptors and γc is required for cytokine signaling via IL-2 and IL-15 [8, 9]. Since T cells and NK cells play a major role in identification and elimination of foreign cells, this mouse strain is ideal for humanization experiments. Transplantation of human HSCs into $Rag2^{-/-}\gamma c^{-/-}$ mice leads to human multi-lineage hematopoiesis and the development of the major functional components of the human adaptive immune system. Human B and T cells, monocytes/macrophages, and dendritic cells are readily detected in lymphoid organs and in the periphery. Humanized mice have been useful in the study of viral pathogenesis and new treatment strategies for human viruses such as HIV-1, human T-lymphotropic virus, Epstein–Barr virus, human cytomegalovirus, and dengue virus [8, 10–15]. In addition, these mice are capable of producing primary human adaptive immune responses such as human antibody and T cell responses against a variety of viral, bacterial, and other antigenic targets [6, 7, 16].

In this chapter we describe the generation of humanized mice through purification of human HSCs, intrahepatic transplantation into newborn BALB/c $Rag2^{-/-}\gamma c^{-/-}$ mice, and verification of successful engraftment through FACS analysis of peripheral blood samples.

2 Materials

2.1 Purification and Culture of Human Hematopoietic Stem Cells

1. Human $CD34^{+}$ Selection Kit (Miltenyi Biotec, Auburn, CA, USA, or Stem Cell Technologies, Vancouver, BC, Canada). We have successfully used both kits.
2. Iscove's Modified Dulbecco's Medium supplemented with 10 % fetal calf serum, 2 % penicillin–streptomycin, and 10 ng/ml each of SCF, IL-3, and IL-6. Filter-sterilize the medium and store at 4 °C.

2.2 Transplantation of BALB/c Rag2$^{-/-}$ $\gamma c^{-/-}$ Mice with Human HSCs

1. BALB/c Rag2$^{-/-}$ $\gamma c^{-/-}$ mice (*see* **Note 1**).
2. 28 gauge insulin syringes.
3. Cultured human HSCs.
4. Iscove's Modified Dulbecco's Medium.

2.3 Bleeding Mice to Screen for Human Cell Engraftment

1. Heating pad.
2. Mouse restraint apparatus (Model TV-150; Braintree scientific Inc., Braintree, MA, USA). This device has a groove across the top. A plunger prevents the mouse from escaping.
3. Scalpel blade (surgical blade stainless steel No. 11).
4. Gauze pads.
5. Styptic powder (Kwik-Stop Styptic Powder with Benzocaine; ARC Laboratories).
6. Heparinized microcapillary tubes (Heparinized Micro-hematocrit capillary tubes; Thermo Fisher Scientific Inc., Waltham, MA, USA).
7. Micropipettor with tips.

2.4 FACS Analysis to Detect and Quantify Human Cell Engraftment

1. Antibodies: hCD45-PE-Cy7 and mCD45-PE (eBioscience, San Diego, CA, USA).
2. 10× ammonium chloride erythrocyte lysing solution: Dissolve 89.9 g NH_4Cl, 10.0 g $KHCO_3$, and 370.0 mg tetrasodium EDTA in 1 liter of ddH_2O. Adjust pH to 7.3. Store at 4 °C in full, tightly closed 50 ml tubes. Dilute to 1× with ddH_2O and use immediately.
3. FACS stain buffer: 1× PBS, 0.1 % BSA, and 0.1 % sodium azide. Store at 4 °C.
4. Fc blocking buffer: Human Gamma Globulin (Jackson Immunoresearch Labs, West Grove, PA, USA), Normal Mouse Serum (Jackson Immunoresearch Labs), 2.4G2 monoclonal antibody to murine CD16/CD32 (BD, Franklin Lakes, NJ, USA). Reconstitute Normal Mouse Serum with 5.0 ml of ddH20. Add 2 ml of Human Gamma Globulin. Add 200 μl of 2.4G2 anti-mouse CD16/CD32. Store at 4 °C.
5. 1 % paraformaldehyde in 1× PBS: Paraformaldehyde does not dissolve effectively in PBS. Prepare a stock of 2 % paraformaldehyde in ddH_2O and a stock of 2× PBS in ddH_2O. Mix these solutions together in equal parts and store at 4 °C.
6. Flow cytometer.
7. FACS tubes.

3 Methods

3.1 Preparation of Human HSCs for Transplantation

1. $CD34^+$ human HSCs are purified from human umbilical cord blood or other sources (*see* **Note 2**) using magnetically labeled antibodies according to the manufacturer's protocol. $CD34^+$ cells are cultured for 40–48 h (*see* **Note 3**) post extraction in IMDM supplemented with 10 % FCS, 1× penicillin/streptomycin, and 10 ng/ml each of IL-3, IL-6, and SCF.
2. Resuspend cells by repeated pipetting, since many cells will be semi-adherent. Count cells using a hemocytometer. Samples used for engrafting mice may be divided to engraft multiple mice.
3. Centrifuge samples for 3 min at 900 × g and discard the supernatant. Resuspend the cell pellet in serum-free IMDM. Approximately 30–50 μl of re-suspended cells is best for an individual mouse injection. Divide the solution into different samples equal to the number of pups that will be engrafted. We use a minimal dose of 250,000 cells per mouse in order to achieve consistent, high-level engraftment (*see* **Note 4**).

3.2 Conditioning Pups for Transplantation

1. 1- to 5-day-old pups (*see* **Note 5**) are conditioned by gamma irradiation at a dose of 350 rads. Wait at least 1 h between irradiation and cell injection. Care must be taken to prevent animals from being exposed to mouse pathogens during transportation and cell injection (*see* **Note 6**).

3.3 Transplantation of Pups with Human HSCs

1. Add 30–50 μl of $CD34^+$ cells in solution into each syringe. The exact volume depends upon the age and size of the pups (*see* **Note 7**). 30 μl is best for 1-day-old pups. Since some volume is retained in the needle after injection, larger volumes are preferable for older pups in order to prevent loss of cells due to retention of liquid in the syringe.
2. Place pups on their backs and stretch out their bodies to allow visualization of the liver. Since pups are albino, the liver is readily visible. Pups are injected with cells in the liver at a depth of 1–2 mm. Greater depths can result in bleeding from the injection site. Following injection keep the syringe inserted for 20 s to prevent cells from being expelled after needle withdrawal. Upon completion of the injection, place the pups back with their mother.

3.4 Bleeding Mice for FACS Analysis

1. Eight weeks post reconstitution, mice should be screened for human cell engraftment. Warm up the mice by placing them in an empty plastic cage on top of a heating pad. Allow at least 5 min for the mice to sufficiently heat up. The mice are warm enough when their movements are rapid and they are breathing quickly.

2. Remove a mouse from the heating cage and place it in the restraint apparatus. Holding the mouse by the tail, gently pull the mouse (tail first) into the apparatus. Pull the tail along the groove in the top of the apparatus, thus pulling the mouse into the apparatus. Push the plunger into the front of the apparatus so that the mouse is held inside (*see* **Note 8**).
3. Locate the veins on the tail and choose one for tail nick bleeding. Using the scalpel, make a small transverse cut across the selected vein. After the mouse begins to bleed, hold the capillary tube horizontally (to avoid forming air bubbles that can lead to clotting) at the cut site and begin collecting blood. When the capillary is full withdraw it (keeping it horizontal) and place the blood sample into an appropriately labeled microfuge tube.
4. Pinch the tail above the cut site to stop the blood flow and wipe away any excess blood. Scoop out a small amount of styptic powder and apply it to the cut site. Allow enough time for clotting to occur. Place the mouse back into its original cage.
5. Eject the blood from the capillary tube using the micropipettor and draw the capillary tube up and out of the microfuge tube as you eject the blood. This technique will prevent the blood from entering back into the capillary.

3.5 Preparing Blood Samples for FACS Analysis

1. Lyse red blood cells by adding 1.4 ml of erythrocyte lysing solution per 100 μl of blood. Incubate at room temperature for 5–10 min. Centrifuge samples at 900 × *g* for 3 min. Discard the supernatant and resuspend the cell pellet in 100 μl of FACS stain buffer.
2. Add 3 μl of Fc blocking buffer and place samples at 4 °C for 15 min (*see* **Note 9**). Add 3 μl of both mCD45-PE and hCD45-PE-Cy7 to each sample and incubate at 4 °C for 30 min. Keep light exposure to a minimum.
3. Add 900 μl of 1 % paraformaldehyde in 1× PBS to each sample. Spin samples at 900 g for 3 min. Dispose of the supernatant and resuspend the pellet in 150 μl of 1× PBS solution. Transfer samples into FACS tubes and analyze by FACS.

4 Notes

1. There are multiple types of immunodeficient mouse strains that support engraftment of human HSCs and multi-lineage hematopoiesis. The original SCID mouse retains natural killer (NK) cell activity and the SCID mutation can result in leaky production of lymphocytes in older mice; both NK cells and T lymphocytes recognize and reject foreign cells. As a result, strains with greater defects in NK and T cell development are now typically used, including Rag2$^{-/-}\gamma c^{-/-}$ mice, NOD/SCID mice,

NOD/SCID $\gamma c^{-/-}$ mice, and Rag1$^{-/-}$ $\gamma c^{-/-}$ mice. Rag2$^{-/-}$ $\gamma c^{-/-}$ mice are commercially available on a C57BL/6 background, but for unknown reasons these animals cannot be effectively engrafted (BALB/c Rag2$^{-/-}$ $\gamma c^{-/-}$ mice work effectively). Excellent reviews are available that explain the phenotype of each mutation, as well as the history of using these strains to produce humanized mice [3, 17].

2. Three main sources are currently employed to obtain HSCs: umbilical cord blood, fetal liver, and mobilized peripheral blood. Magnetic separation techniques are commonly employed to purify CD34^{+} cells. Umbilical cord blood is most readily available, but this source yields a low number of cells, at most 1×10^6. Relatively fewer mice can be engrafted per sample due to lower yields. Fetal liver samples have ethical constraints and few suppliers exist, but these samples yield more cells. Fetal liver samples commonly yield greater than 20×10^6 cells. We have no experience using mobilized peripheral blood and this source is rarely used to produce humanized mice [18, 19].

3. CD34^{+} cells are cultured for 40–48 h in order to obtain maximum expansion of the hematopoietic stem cell population while preventing differentiation of the stem cells. There is no method currently available to culture HSCs without eventual differentiation and loss of potency for engraftment. Density of cells is critical for expansion during culture. Denser cell cultures grow more efficiently than cultures that are less dense. We culture cells in 48-well plates since that provides the appropriate cell density for most umbilical cord blood-derived samples.

4. The number of CD34^{+} HSCs to inject varies considerably in the literature. In the original paper by Traggiai et al. showing HSC engraftment in Rag2$^{-/-}$ $\gamma c^{-/-}$ mice, they found engraftment with as few as 3.8×10^4 CD34^{+} HSCs [8]. We typically use at least 2.5×10^5 cells per mouse to achieve consistent, high-level engraftment. Some researchers use up to $1–2 \times 10^6$ cells per mouse [20].

5. Several experiments have shown that age of mice at the time of engraftment has an impact on the level of engraftment achieved. We have found that engraftment levels are superior when Rag2$^{-/-}$ $\gamma c^{-/-}$ pups are less than 5 days of age at the time of irradiation and transplantation. Attempts to engraft older Rag2$^{-/-}$ $\gamma c^{-/-}$ mice result in lower levels of engraftment. Different mouse strains can show effective engraftment with older mice (e.g., NOD/SCID $\gamma c^{-/-}$), but in some cases different conditioning techniques were used [19, 21–23].

6. Immunodeficient mice are housed in specific pathogen-free facilities because they are unable to defend against various types of infections. They are often given antibiotics in their

drinking water in order to prevent bacterial infection. When preparing mice for irradiation, they often have to leave the animal facility; therefore, great care must be taken to keep the animals pathogen-free while in transit so as to avoid contaminating the colony.

7. Intrahepatic injection into newborn mice can be technically challenging. BALB/c mice are albino and hence the liver is readily visible. We typically inject a volume of 30–50 μl of cells per mouse. However, we find that the volume used for cell injection must be smaller for 1-day-old pups; if not the inoculated cells can exit the injection site after withdrawing the needle due to pressure accumulated during injection. For smaller pups, we use an injection volume of 30 μl. Allow the needle to remain in place for 20 s to ensure that the cells will not be expelled from the mouse.
8. Be careful not to catch the mouse's feet between the plunger and the wall of the apparatus. Do not let go of the tail or the mouse may pull the tail inside. Animals can sometimes bury their heads underneath their bodies and suffocate, so make sure that the head stays up for access to fresh air.
9. FACS analysis using cells from chimeric animals is more complicated than using cells from a single organism due to the requirement to block nonspecific antibody binding to both human and mouse cells. We perform initial workup experiments with FACS antibodies on pure mouse blood or pure human blood to verify the accuracy of the staining. We block nonspecific staining by using a combination mouse/human Fc block consisting of anti-mouse CD16/CD32, human gamma globulin, and normal mouse serum (*see* Subheading 2). We typically use mouse monoclonal antibodies for FACS staining and we rarely detect background or cross-species staining.

Acknowledgments

This work was supported by a Mentoring Environment Grant from Brigham Young University.

References

1. Bosma GC, Custer RP, Bosma MJ (1983) A severe combined immunodeficiency mutation in the mouse. Nature 301(5900):527–530
2. Brehm MA, Shultz LD, Greiner DL (2010) Humanized mouse models to study human diseases. Curr Opin Endocrinol Diabetes Obes 17(2):120–125
3. Shultz LD, Ishikawa F, Greiner DL (2007) Humanized mice in translational biomedical research. Nat Rev Immunol 7:118–130
4. Pearson T, Greiner DL, Shultz LD (2008) Humanized SCID mouse models for biomedical research. Curr Top Microbiol Immunol 324:25–51

5. Goldstein H (2008) Summary of presentations at the NIH/NIAID New Humanized Rodent Models 2007 Workshop. AIDS Res Ther 5:3
6. Goldman JP, Blundell MP, Lopes L, Kinnon C, Di Santo JP, Thrasher AJ (1998) Enhanced human cell engraftment in mice deficient in RAG2 and the common cytokine receptor gamma chain. Br J Haematol 103(2):335–342
7. Mazurier F, Gan OI, McKenzie JL, Doedens M, Dick JE (1999) A novel immunodeficient mouse model–RAG2 x common cytokine receptor gamma chain double mutants–requiring exogenous cytokine administration for human hematopoietic stem cell engraftment. J Interferon Cytokine Res 19(5):533–541
8. Traggiai E, Chicha L, Mazzucchelli L, Bronz L, Piffaretti JC, Lanzavecchia A, Manz MG (2004) Development of a human adaptive immune system in cord blood cell-transplanted mice. Science 304:104–107
9. Baenziger S, Tussiwand R, Schlaepfer E, Mazzucchelli L, Heikenwalder M, Kurrer MO, Behnke S, Frey J, Oxenius A, Joller H, Aguzzi A, Manz MG, Speck RF (2006) Disseminated and sustained HIV infection in CD34+ cord blood cell-transplanted Rag2−/−gc−/− mice. Proc Natl Acad Sci U S A 103:15951–15956
10. Berges BK, Wheat WH, Palmer B, Connick E, Akkina R (2006) HIV-1 infection and CD4 T cell depletion in the humanized Rag2−/−gc−/− (RAG-hu) mouse model. Retrovirology 3:76
11. Berges BK, Rowan MR (2011) The utility of the new generation of humanized mice to study HIV-1 infection: transmission, prevention, pathogenesis, and treatment. Retrovirology 8:65
12. Kuruvilla JG, Troyer RM, Devi S, Akkina R (2007) Dengue virus infection and immune response in humanized Rag2$^{-/-}$gc$^{-/-}$ (RAG-hu) mice. Virol 369:143–152
13. Smith MS, Goldman DC, Bailey AS, Pfaffle DL, Kreklywich CN, Spencer DB, Othieno FA, Streblow DN, Garcia JV, Fleming WH, Nelson JA, Smith MS (2012) Granulocyte-colony stimulating factor reactivates human cytomegalovirus in a latently infected humanized mouse model. Cell Host Microbe 8:284–291
14. Banerjee P, Tripp A, Lairmore MD, Crawford L, Sieburg M, Ramos J, Harrington W Jr, Beilke MA, Feuer G (2010) Adult T cell leukemia/lymphoma development in HTLV-1-infected humanized SCID mice. Blood 115:2640–2648
15. Berges BK, Akkina SR, Remling L, Akkina R (2010) Humanized Rag2(−/−)gammac(−/−) (RAG-hu) mice can sustain long-term chronic HIV-1 infection lasting more than a year. Virol 397:100–103
16. Chicha L, Tussiwand R, Traggiai E, Mazzucchelli L, Bronz L, Piffaretti JC, Lanzavecchia A, Manz MG (2005) Human adaptive immune system Rag2−/−gamma(c)−/− mice. Ann N Y Acad Sci 1044:236–243
17. Manz MG (2007) Human-hemato-lymphoid-system mice: opportunities and challenges. Immunity 26:537–541
18. Lang J, Weiss N, Freed BM, Torres RM, Pelanda R (2011) Generation of hematopoietic humanized mice in the newborn BALB/c-Rag2(null)Il2rγ(null) mouse model: a multivariable optimization approach. Clin Immunol 140:102–116
19. Shultz LD, Lyons BL, Burzenski LM, Gott B, Chen X, Chaleff S, Kotb M, Gillies SD, King M, Mangada J, Greiner DL, Handgretinger R (2005) Human lymphoid and myeloid cell development in NOD/LtSz-scid IL2R gamma null mice engrafted with mobilized human hemopoietic stem cells. J Immun 174: 6477–6489
20. Kwant-Mitchell A, Ashkar AA, Rosenthal KL (2009) Mucosal innate and adaptive immune responses against HSV-2 in a humanized mouse model. J Virol 83:10664–10676
21. Brehm MA, Cuthbert A, Yang C, Miller DM, DiIorio P, Laning J, Burzenski L, Gott B, Foreman O, Kavirayani A, Herlihy M, Rossini AA, Shultz LD, Greiner DL (2010) Parameters for establishing humanized mouse models to study human immunity: analysis of human hematopoietic stem cell engraftment in three immunodeficient strains of mice bearing the IL2rgamma(null) mutation. Clin Immunol 135:84–98
22. Pearson T, Shultz LD, Miller D, King M, Laning J, Fodor W, Cuthbert A, Burzenski L, Gott B, Lyons B, Foreman O, Rossini AA, Greiner DL (2008) Non-obese diabetic-recombination activating gene-1 (NOD-Rag 1(null)) interleukin (IL)-2 receptor common gamma chain (IL 2 rgamma(null)) null mice: a radioresistant model for human lymphohaematopoietic engraftment. Clin Exp Immunol 154:270–284
23. Rozemuller H, Knaan-Shanzer S, Hagenbeek A, van Bloois L, Storm G, Martens AC (2004) Enhanced engraftment of human cells in RAG2/gammac double-knockout mice after treatment with CL2MDP liposomes. Exp Hematol 32:1118–1125

Chapter 3

Isolation, Culture, and Functional Evaluation of Bone Marrow-Derived Macrophages

Beckley K. Davis

Abstract

Macrophages are cellular components of the immune system that are essential for responding to pathogens, initiating inflammation, and maintaining tissue homeostasis. Isolation, culture, and functional characterization of bone marrow-derived macrophages from mice are exceptionally powerful techniques used to examine aspects of macrophage biology in vitro. These cells can be used to study effector functions, such as phagocytosis, cytokine secretion, oxidative burst, migration, antigen processing and presentation, in the context of wild-type, gene-ablated, and/or transgenic mice. The quantity, purity, and ease of culture of these cells enhance their utility for primary cell cultures. This chapter outlines protocols used to generate, quantitate, and functionally evaluate macrophages derived from bone marrow precursor cells.

Key words Bone marrow, Macrophage, Inflammation, Cytokine, Phagocytosis, ELISA, Flow cytometry

1 Introduction

The innate immune system in metazoans recognizes invariant microbial structures, such as pathogen-associated molecular patterns (PAMPs) and host-derived danger- or damage-associated molecular patterns (DAMPs). Activation of receptors associated with these molecules leads to changes in cell morphology, effector function, and cytokine production. These changes can have both beneficial and detrimental outcomes for the host, as well as have profound effects on shaping the ensuing adaptive immune response. Cells of the innate immune system include granulocytes, monocytes, macrophages, and dendritic cells.

The in vivo role of macrophages is being reevaluated as current research uncovers unexpected biological roles. These cells and their associated processes have been linked to many diverse pathologies, including infection, inflammation, allergy and asthma, metabolic disorders, and tumorigenesis [1–4]. Mouse macrophages have

Irving C. Allen (ed.), *Mouse Models of Innate Immunity: Methods and Protocols*, Methods in Molecular Biology, vol. 1031, DOI 10.1007/978-1-62703-481-4_3, © Springer Science+Business Media, LLC 2013

become a cognate animal model for the study of human macrophage biology and disease.

Macrophages represent a heterogenous population of functionally, developmentally, and phenotypically distinct cells. Their functional plasticity, in part, relates to their many tissue-specific roles in host physiology, for example Kupffer cells of the liver are vastly different from microglia cells of the brain. Broadly, these cells are capable of phagocytosis and the generation of effector molecules such as cytokines, chemokines, and antimicrobial effector molecules. However, tissue-specific phenotypes exist [5]. Functional characterization of tissue-specific macrophages is hampered by the low frequencies of these cells and the technically challenging, cost-prohibitive protocols for the isolation of these cells. Nevertheless, generation of high-yield and relatively homogenous populations of macrophages is a necessary prerequisite for research of macrophage biology.

Bone marrow-derived macrophages provide a tractable system to study primary cell function. These cells are easily cultured and manipulated, retain their biological functions, are viable for 7–10 days, can be transfected, and are used widely in the scientific community. In the bone marrow, granulocyte/macrophage colony-stimulating factor (GM-CSF), macrophage colony-stimulating factor (M-CSF), and interleukin-3 (IL-3) stimulate granulocyte–monocyte colony-forming units to mature into monocyte precursors [6]. These precursor cells leave the bone marrow and can further mature into either macrophages (via M-CSF) or dendritic cells (via GM-CSF and interleukin-4), both of which migrate from systemic circulation into peripheral tissues.

Macrophages that reside in peripheral tissues can be isolated as well [7]. A common technique for the isolation of peripheral tissue-associated macrophages is positive selection using immunomagnetic methods. These protocols are costly and the relative yield of macrophages is low. In comparison, large numbers of thioglycollate-elicited macrophages can be isolated by lavage of the mouse peritoneum [8], notwithstanding these cells are typically activated and may not be amenable to downstream applications. Non-elicited peritoneum exudate cells are a mixed population. However, these cells are considered naïve and have been used ex vivo [9]. Nonetheless, the purity of these cells must be addressed either by differential staining or flow cytometry. Commonly used transformed macrophage-like mouse cell lines, such as RAW264.7 and J774.1 cells [10], can be used in parallel with the primary cell culture outlined in this chapter. Likewise monocyte-derived macrophages from peripheral blood mononuclear cells from human leukopaks [11] or human transformed cell lines, such as THP-1 or U937, can be used comparatively to assess macrophage biology in humans.

The protocols outlined below are commonly used to assess macrophage function. Other experimental protocols exist and slight modifications to the protocols outlined here can be used to generate macrophages from bone marrow. These methods allow for the generation of large quantities of macrophages that can be readily used in research. Bone marrow-derived macrophages can be used in conjunction with tissue-specific macrophages, species-specific macrophages, or transformed cell lines.

2 Materials

2.1 Harvest

1. Personal protective equipment, including but not limited to laboratory coat, gloves, and goggles (*see* **Note 1**).
2. Age- and sex-matched C57Bl/6 mice.
3. Laminar flow hood.
4. Surgical instruments: Forceps and scissors or bone cutters.
5. 20–27 G needles.
6. 3 or 5 cc syringes.
7. 100 μm cell strainer.
8. Hemocytometer.
9. Light microscope.

2.2 Culturing

1. Tissue culture incubator.
2. Tissue culture centrifuge.
3. Sterile and pyrogen-free PBS (without Ca^{++} and Mg^{++}).
4. Hank's Balanced Salt Solution.
5. Trypsin:EDTA.
6. Penicillin (10,000 U/ml)/streptomycin (10,000 μg/ml) solution.
7. Certified low-endotoxin fetal bovine serum (FBS).
8. L-glutamine solution (29.2 mg/ml).
9. Sodium pyruvate solution (100 mM).
10. Nonessential amino acids solution.
11. Macrophage media: DMEM supplemented with 20 % L929 conditioned media, 10 % heat-inactivated FBS, 1 % L-glutamine, 1 % sodium pyruvate, 1 % nonessential amino acids, and 1 % penicillin/streptomycin.
12. L929 (ATCC no CCL-1) conditioned media: Grow cells to 90 % confluency in DMEM supplemented with 10 % heat-inactivated FBS, 1 % L-glutamine, 1 % sodium pyruvate, 1 % nonessential amino acids, and 1 % penicillin/streptomycin. Media should be filtered through a 0.45 μm filter and stored at −20 °C until use. L929 cells are an inexpensive source of

M-CSF. Alternatively commercially available M-CSF can be used at 10^4 U/ml.

13. Tissue culture-treated plates: 100×20 mm; 150×25 mm; 6-well plate; 12-well plate; 24-well plate.
14. Ultralow bind non-treated culture plates.
15. Pipettes; pipettors; and pipette aids.
16. Tubes: 1.5 ml; 15 ml BD Falcon™ conical tubes; 50 ml BD Falcon™ conical tubes.

2.3 Functional Assays

1. Cell scraper.
2. Diff-Quick staining reagents (Fisher Scientific).
3. Microscope slides.
4. Flow cytometer (Accuri C6, BD FACScan, or an equivalent).
5. Anti-F4/80-FITC antibody.
6. Anti-CD11b (Mac-1)-PE antibody.
7. Isotype control antibody.
8. ELISA plate reader (Molecular Devices SpectraMax or an equivalent).
9. ELISA kits: IL-1β; IL-6; TNF-α; and IFN-β.

3 Methods

3.1 Isolation

1. C57Bl/6 mice from specific pathogen-free housing should be used (*see* **Note 2**). Euthanize mice according to current Institutional Animal Care and Use Committee (IACUC) guidelines. Animals should be sex matched for minor histocompatibility antigens. We use 8–12-week-old donor mice for all of our experiments.
2. Prepare one mouse at a time on a dissection tray (*see* **Note 3**). Spray down the carcass with 70 % ethanol to sterilize the field.
3. Pin the carcass down with the ventral side facing up with dissecting pins or large-gauge needles.
4. Apply forceps to the skin anterior to the urethral opening. With scissors, cut the skin along the ventral midline from the groin to the chin, carefully avoiding the underlying musculature.
5. Next, with scissors, make an incision from the start of the first incision caudally to the ankle on both sides of the animal. Carefully peel the skin off the appendages to the ankle joint (*see* **Note 4**).
6. Remove tissue from the legs with scissors and dissect the leg away from the body.

7. Denude the remaining soft tissue from the pelvic and femoral bones, and separate proximal to the knee joint and the pelvic girdle (*see* **Note 5**).
8. Immerse the dissected femurs in 70 % ethanol for 1 min.
9. Wash twice in 1× DPBS containing 1 % penicillin (500–1,000 U/ml)/streptomycin (500–1,1000 μg/ml).
10. While supporting the femur with forceps, use a 25 G (*see* **Note 6**) needle fitted to either a 3 or a 5 cc syringe filled with 2 ml of 1× DPBS (*see* **Note 7**), and carefully insert the needle into the bone marrow cavity. Gently expel the bone marrow from the bone with a jet of liquid directed into a 15 ml screw top tube containing 5 ml of pre-warmed 1× DPBS. Repeat and articulate the needle along the bone shaft to ensure that a majority of the bone marrow has been evacuated from the cavity. Pass the bone marrow through a 0.45 μm cell strainer to remove any debris.
11. Centrifuge cells for 10 min at 300×*g* at 10 °C. Discard the supernatant.
12. Count bone marrow cells with a hemocytometer and adjust the cells to a density of 5×10^6 cells/ml in macrophage media.

3.2 Culturing

1. Add 2 to 5×10^5 cells to a sterile tissue culture (100×15 cm) or petri dish (*see* **Note 8**).
2. Incubate for 6–7 days (*see* **Note 9**) in a 5 % CO_2 humidified tissue culture incubator. Check cells daily (*see* **Note 10**), and add fresh media (5 ml) every 2–3 days.
3. On day 6 or 7, discard the media in the tissue culture dish and wash the adherent cells once with 1× DPBS. Add 5–7 ml of 0.05 % trypsin–EDTA solution and incubate for 15–20 min at 37 °C (*see* **Note 11**).
4. Dislodge the cells with gentle washing using a pipette aid.
5. Wash the cells by centrifugation for 5 min at 300×*g* and resuspend in macrophage media without L929 conditioned media.
6. $2\text{–}6 \times 10^7$ macrophages can be obtained from a single mouse (two femurs).

3.3 Phenotyping

1. Resuspend $1\text{–}5 \times 10^5$ cells in 100 μl of 1× DPBS supplemented with 2 % FBS and 2 mm EDTA in a 1.5 ml tube (*see* **Note 12**).
2. Add fluorescently labeled anti-F4/80, Mac-1 antibodies, and isotype controls (*see* **Note 13**) and incubate on ice in the dark for 30 min.
3. Wash 2× with 1× DPBS supplemented with 2 % FCS.
4. Resuspend cells in 500 μl of wash buffer.

5. Analyze the cells by flow cytometry. Macrophages should be positive for both F4/80 and CD11b. Cell purity should range from 90 to 99 % double-positive cells.
6. Bright field microscopy can also be used to evaluate macrophage morphology, phagocytosis, and oxidative bursts [15].
7. To perform these assays, grow 1×10^5 cells on glass coverslips in 6-well tissue culture plates.
8. Perform differential staining with Diff-Quick™ as per the manufacturer's suggested protocol (*see* **Note 14**).
9. Visualize under bright field microscopy.

3.4 Cytokine Secretion (See Note 15)

1. Stimulate cells with 10 ng–10 μg/ml of LPS; 0.1–1.0 μg/ml of Pam3CSK4; 10^8/ml of heat-killed *Listeria monocytogenes*; 10 ng–10 μg/ml of flagellin; 10–10 μg/ml of Poly I:C; 0.25–10 μg/ml of ssRNA; or 5 μM of unmethylated CpG (*see* **Note 16**). These reagents should be diluted in pyrogen-free water or saline.
2. Incubate cells with TLR agonists for 6–8 h at 37 °C and 5 % CO_2 in a humidified tissue culture incubator (*see* **Note 17**).
3. Harvest tissue culture supernatants by centrifugation at $500 \times g$ for 5 min. Transfer the supernatant to a new 1.5 ml tube. Use immediately for cytokine secretion or store samples at −80 °C for later use.
4. The supernatants produced above may be assessed using enzyme-linked immunosorbent assay (ELISA) for cytokine production. We have routinely assayed IL-1β, IL-6, IL-18, TNF-α, and IFN-β from bone marrow-derived macrophages stimulated with TLR agonists.

3.5 Phagocytosis

1. Grow $0.5–1.0 \times 10^6$ bone marrow-derived macrophage cells on glass coverslips in 6-well plates in bone marrow macrophage media overnight.
2. The following day, aspirate media, add fresh bone marrow media with either fluorescently labeled heat-killed *E. coli* (1–100 bacteria/cell) or zymosan (1–100 particles/cell) (*see* **Note 18**). Incubate the cells at 37 °C in 5 % CO_2 for 15–60 min (*see* **Note 19**).
3. Wash cells five times with 1 ml of 1× DPBS supplemented with 2 % fetal calf serum to remove non-phagocytized particles.
4. Fix cells with 1 ml of 4 % paraformaldehyde in 1× DPBS for 15 min (*see* **Note 20**).
5. Wash the cells three times with 1 ml of 1× DPBS.
6. Permeabilize cells with 1 ml of 1× DPBS supplemented with 2 % fetal calf serum and 0.5 % Triton X-100 (*see* **Note 21**).

7. Wash two times with 1 ml of 1× DPBS.
8. Add 1 μg/ml of fluorescently labeled phalloidin in 1 ml of 1 × DPBS and incubate in the dark for 30 min.
9. Wash the cells three times with 1 ml of 1× DPBS.
10. Blot the coverslips dry with an absorbent towel.
11. Mount the coverslip on a slide with mounting media containing 4′,6-diamidino-2-phenylindole, dihydrochloride (DAPI) and *SlowFade*® Gold Antifade.
12. Analyze on a fluorescent microscope (*see* **Note 22**).

4 Notes

1. It is imperative that all solutions remain sterile and pyrogen-free. Bone marrow-derived macrophages are exceptionally sensitive to bacterial moieties. If possible, all manipulations should be carried out in a laminar flow hood using aseptic techniques. The generation of bone marrow-derived macrophages from novel, transgenic, or gene ablation mice may require individual optimization. We have successfully used these protocols using wild-type mice and several novel mouse strains [9, 12–14].
2. We use C57Bl/6 mice to derive macrophages; however, other groups have used commonly available inbred strains using similar protocols. In all cases we exclusively use mice housed in specific pathogen-free facilities to minimize the activation status of macrophages.
3. Disposable dissecting trays can be fashioned out of Styrofoam.
4. In addition to bone marrow-derived cells, tissue-specific macrophages can be harvested in parallel. Tissue-derived cells can be harvested from diverse sources, including the spleen, liver, lung, and intestine. Other immunologically relevant tissues such as spleen, lymph nodes, and thymus can also be harvested at this time to assay different cellular components, making full use of the experimental animal.
5. Tibia bones are also a source for bone marrow and can be processed in an analogous manner to increase the yield per mouse of bone marrow precursor cells. The tibias should be separated at the ankle joint.
6. We have used 20–27 G needles to irrigate femurs. Smaller gauge needles will be easier to use for tibial bone marrow evacuations.
7. We have used different isotonic solutions (1× DBPS, DMEM, and HBSS) to irrigate the bone marrow cavity with no decrease in cell numbers, viability, or biological function.

8. We have used both treated and non-treated tissue culture plasticware to cultivate bone marrow-derived macrophages. We prefer to use treated plasticware to avoid possible confusion while growing different cell types. As a result of using treated tissue culture plasticware, bone marrow-derived macrophages adhere tightly to these dishes and may require physical dissociation with a cell scraper or prolonged treatment with trypsin:EDTA solution.
9. We have noticed slight variability in bone marrow-derived macrophage growth and maturation, possibly due to variability of growth factors (M-CSF) in L929 conditioned media.
10. Daily inspection of cells allows for visual confirmation of cell growth, adherence, and possibility of contamination.
11. Bone marrow macrophages can adhere tightly to tissue culture-treated plasticware and may require increased incubation time with 0.05 % trypsin:EDTA, increased concentration of trypsin:EDTA solution, or mechanical detachment with a cell scraper.
12. For higher throughput analysis, 96-well round-bottom tissue culture plates can be used in place of 1.5 ml tubes.
13. We have used many different fluorophores and antibody sources. It is imperative that the fluorophores do not overlap in emission spectra and are compatible with the flow cytometer laser.
14. Differential staining by Romanowsky staining (Diff-Quik™) can provide an easy means by which cells can be identified and their relative percentages obtained.
15. The day before the experiment, harvest the bone marrow-derived macrophages and plate in 6-, 12- or 24-well tissue culture plates at densities of $0.5–1.0 \times 10^6$ in 3 ml, $3–5 \times 10^5$ in 2 ml, or $0.5–2 \times 10^5$ cells in 1 ml of media, respectively.
16. We have used TLR agonists from Invivogen; other vendors such as Sigma and Invitrogen provide similar products.
17. We have seen sufficient cytokine secretion (IL-1β, IL-6, TNF-α, and IFN-β) in response to TLR stimulation in bone marrow-derived macrophages. Assays may require additional incubation times depending upon the stimulus and the biological readout. Also, it may be necessary to dilute the samples in order to fall within the linear range of the assay.
18. Different substrates can be used to effectively determine relative phagocytosis indexes. Light microscopy with differential staining can be used instead of fluorescent microscopy to determine phagocytosis of either bacteria or yeast.
19. The rate of phagocytosis may be variable depending on individual preparations of bone marrow-derived macrophages, their activation status, and the substrates used.

20. Other methods of fixation can be used. Aldehydes are the most common fixative. Care must be used when dealing with either paraformaldehyde or glutaraldehyde as both chemicals are suspected carcinogens. 100 % Ice-cold methanol precipitation can be used with satisfactory results.
21. Permeabilization is accomplished by the addition of detergent; we have used other detergents, such as saponin, with similar results.
22. Flow cytometry can be used to analyze the relative amount of phagocytosis of bacteria [9].

References

1. Mège JL, Mehraj V, Capo C (2011) Macrophage polarization and bacterial infections. Curr Opin Infect Dis 24(3): 230–234
2. Bloemen K, Verstraelen S, Van Den Heuvel R, Witters H, Nelissen I, Schoeters G (2007) The allergic cascade: review of the most important molecules in the asthmatic lung. Immunol Lett 113(1):6–18
3. Chawla A, Nguyen KD, Goh YP (2011) Macrophage-mediated inflammation in metabolic disease. Nat Rev Immunol 11(11): 738–749
4. Biswas SK, Mantovani A (2010) Macrophage plasticity and interaction with lymphocyte subsets: cancer as a paradigm. Nat Immunol 11(10):889–896
5. Karp CL, Murray PJ (2012) Non-canonical alternatives: what a macrophage is 4. J Exp Med 209(3):427–431
6. Geissmann F, Manz MG, Jung S, Sieweke MH, Merad M, Ley K (2010) Development of monocytes, macrophages, and dendritic cells. Science 327(5966):656–661
7. Morio LA, Chiu H, Sprowles KA, Laskin DL (2000) Functional heterogeneity of rat hepatic and alveolar macrophages: effects of chronic ethanol administration. J Leukoc Biol 68(5):614–620
8. McElvania Tekippe E, Allen IC, Hulseberg PD, Sullivan JT, McCann JR, Sandor M, Braunstein M, Ting JP (2010) Granuloma formation and host defense in chronic Mycobacterium tuberculosis infection requires PYCARD/ASC but not NLRP3 or caspase-1. PLoS One 5(8):e12320
9. Wen H, Lei Y, Eun SY, Ting JP (2010) Plexin-A4-semaphorin 3A signaling is required for toll-like receptor- and sepsis-induced cytokine storm. J Exp Med 207(13):2943–2957
10. Mesquita FS, Thomas M, Sachse M, Santos AJ, Figueira R, Holden DW (2012) The Salmonella deubiquitinase SseL inhibits selective autophagy of cytosolic aggregates. PLoS Pathog 8(6):e1002743
11. Sharif O, Bolshakov VN, Raines S, Newham P, Perkins ND (2007) Transcriptional profiling of the LPS induced NF-κB response in macrophages. BMC Immunol 8:1
12. Allen IC, Wilson JE, Schneider M, Lich JD, Roberts RA, Arthur JC, Woodford RM, Davis BK, Uronis JM, Herfarth HH, Jobin C, Rogers AB, Ting JP (2012) NLRP12 suppresses colon inflammation and tumorigenesis through the negative regulation of noncanonical NF-κB signaling. Immunity 36(5):742–754
13. Allen IC, TeKippe EM, Woodford RM, Uronis JM, Holl EK, Rogers AB, Herfarth HH, Jobin C, Ting JP (2010) The NLRP3 inflammasome functions as a negative regulator of tumorigenesis during colitis-associated cancer. J Exp Med 207(5):1045–1056
14. Allen IC, Moore CB, Schneider M, Lei Y, Davis BK, Scull MA, Gris D, Roney KE, Zimmermann AG, Bowzard JB, Ranjan P, Monroe KM, Pickles RJ, Sambhara S, Ting JP (2011) NLRX1 protein attenuates inflammatory responses to infection by interfering with the RIG-I-MAVS and TRAF6-NF-κB signaling pathways. Immunity 34(6):854–865
15. Selinummi J, Ruusuvuori P, Podolsky I, Ozinsky A, Gold E, Yli-Harja O, Aderem A, Shmulevich I (2009) Bright field microscopy as an alternative to whole cell fluorescence in automated analysis of macrophage images. PLoS One 4(10):e7497

Chapter 4

Collecting Resident or Thioglycollate-Elicited Peritoneal Macrophages

Monika Schneider

Abstract

Peritoneal macrophages are invaluable for gaining an understanding of innate immune responses due to their physiological relevance. These macrophages can be harvested from the peritoneum to give a resident population or can be elicited through the use of thioglycollate. This chapter describes how to collect each type of macrophage.

Key words Primary macrophages, Ex vivo, Innate immunity

1 Introduction

Macrophages are one of the first cell types to respond to infection or injury of the host tissue. Resident macrophages produce cytokines and chemokines that attract other cells, including neutrophils and additional macrophages. Depending on the stimuli, macrophages can initiate a proinflammatory response, apoptosis, motility programs, and phagocytosis. All of these responses can be used as readouts and are useful in assessing the role of pathogenic genes or proteins. There are four commonly utilized macrophage preparations: primary resident macrophages, thioglycollate-elicited macrophages, bone marrow-derived macrophages, and in vitro macrophage cell lines. However, there are caveats to each of the available macrophage models. Tissue-resident macrophages yield results most similar to those in in vivo experiments, but are only present in small numbers, making it difficult to obtain enough for use in experiments. Macrophages that are elicited or derived using cytokines can be obtained in high numbers, but have an activated profile, which can often skew results. Bone marrow-derived macrophages present a high yield, but are less physiologically relevant. Macrophage-like or monocycte-like cell lines can be easy to work with and can be grown to large quantities, but they will often contain a mutation that will confound results. Therefore, it is

Irving C. Allen (ed.), *Mouse Models of Innate Immunity: Methods and Protocols*, Methods in Molecular Biology, vol. 1031, DOI 10.1007/978-1-62703-481-4_4, © Springer Science+Business Media, LLC 2013

important to have a macrophage cell type available that offers a high yield of cells with minimal animal expenditure while still maintaining biological relevance.

2 Materials

1. Mice (male or female; 8–10 weeks old).
2. 3 % thioglycollate medium (Sigma) in ddH_2O, autoclaved.
3. Needles: 18, 26, and 30G.
4. Syringes: 5 and 10cc.
5. 70 % ethanol.
6. DMEM (high glucose), containing 10 % FBS, 1× L-glutamine, 1× nonessential amino acids, 1 % penicillin/streptomycin.
7. 1× PBS.
8. Forceps.
9. Blunt-end scissors.
10. 15 mL polypropylene conical tubes.
11. Hemacytometer.
12. Trypan blue (Sigma).
13. Plates for cell culture (tissue culture treated).

3 Methods

3.1 Thioglycollate-Elicited Peritoneal Macrophages (See Note 1)

1. Fill a 5cc syringe with 3 % thioglycollate (*see* **Note 2**). Attach a 30G needle and inject 1 mL of the solution into the peritoneal cavity of each mouse (*see* **Note 3**).
2. Return the mouse to its cage and allow the immune response to proceed for 5–7 days.
3. Euthanize mice by CO_2 asphyxiation, following institutional guidelines.
4. Pin down each foot of the mouse to a dissecting board, with the abdomen facing up. Using the forceps, pull up the skin above the sternum and make an incision. Use care to avoid piercing the peritoneum/abdominal cavity.
5. Using blunt-end scissors, gently separate the skin from the thoracic cavity and make a horizontal incision down the body of the mouse, and then an incision down the left and the right legs of the mouse.
6. Pull the skin away from peritoneum and pin it down to the dissecting board, keeping skin taut.
7. Fill a 5cc syringe with 1× PBS and attach a 26G needle.

8. At the lower right base of the peritoneal cavity, insert the needle and inject 5 mL of PBS. Be careful not to nick any internal organs, particularly the intestines.
9. Massage the inflated cavity to dislodge cells. Wait at least 30 s before harvesting.
10. Attach an 18G needle to an empty 5cc syringe. Insert the needle on the lower right side of the peritoneum, being careful not to nick any organs. Gently suction peritoneal lavage into the syringe (*see* **Note 4**).
11. Remove the needle from the syringe and transfer the lavage to a 15 mL conical tube. Keep on ice.
12. Centrifuge the cells at 300 × *g* for 5 min.
13. Resuspend cells in 10 mL of supplemented DMEM and count the cells using a hemocytometer and trypan blue stain. Centrifuge the cells again at 300 × *g* for 5 min and resuspend in supplemented DMEM at the desired concentration.

3.2 Resident Peritoneal Macrophages

1. Follow Subheading 3.1, **steps 3–12**.
2. Resuspend the cells in 3 mL of supplemented DMEM and count using a hemocytometer and trypan blue stain. Centrifuge again at 300 × *g* for 5 min and resuspend at the desired concentration (*see* **Note 5**).
3. Plate the cells in a 12-well tissue culture-treated dish and incubate overnight at 37 °C for adherence.
4. Remove non-adherent cells and replace with fresh supplemented DMEM. Cells can be used immediately or within the next 48 h.

4 Notes

1. Ensure that you have secured appropriate institutional approval before beginning animal experiments.
2. Thioglycollate becomes more potent at eliciting macrophages over time. When the solution is first made, it will be a light green/blue color and will quickly change to a light pink or purple color. The thioglycollate solution is most effective when it is a light brown color due to the breakdown of various antigens and sugars. We recommend that you allow the thioglycollate solution to age at least 1 month before using. Keep the solution at room temperature in the dark to avoid contamination.
3. To avoid hitting any internal organs, inject the mouse right of center, approximately level with the knee and about 1 cm left of where the leg meets the torso.

4. There should be a pocket of liquid in the peritoneal cavity on each side of the mouse. This area is the easiest spot to insert the needle without hitting organs. Switch sides when you are no longer able to draw lavage out without also drawing up intestines. From 5 mL of PBS, the lavage yield should be about 3–4 mL.
5. The resident cells in the peritoneal lavage are composed of about 60 % macrophages. Therefore, you will be discarding about 40 % of the cells after the macrophages adhere. Adjust the plating concentration accordingly.

Chapter 5

Quantification and Visualization of Neutrophil Extracellular Traps (NETs) from Murine Bone Marrow-Derived Neutrophils

Linda Vong, Philip M. Sherman, and Michael Glogauer

Abstract

Neutrophils are one of the first cells to respond to an inflammatory stimulus, and are equipped with an assortment of antimicrobial and proteolytic enzymes to disarm and degrade bacterial pathogens. A novel mechanism of bacterial trapping, termed neutrophil extracellular traps (NETs), was recently described whereby neutrophils were shown to cast out web-like structures of chromatin, capturing and immobilizing invading pathogens. Herein we describe protocols to isolate murine bone marrow-derived neutrophils, and spectrophotometrically quantify, immunolabel, and visualize NET structures in vitro.

Key words Neutrophil extracellular trap, Bone marrow neutrophil, Nucleic acid stain, Histone H3, Elastase, Fluorescence microscopy

1 Introduction

Neutrophils mature in the bone marrow, where they synthesize and package enzymes and antimicrobial proteins into an assortment of granules [1]. The formation of neutrophil extracellular traps (NET), a type of novel cell death, is characterized by the externalization of web-like strands of decondensed chromatin (DNA and histones) that is highly decorated with antimicrobial and proteolytic enzymes [2–4]. Such a defined composition can be utilized to specifically label for NETs.

Unlike human bone marrow, mouse bone marrow contains a large number of functionally competent neutrophils, which survive much longer ex vivo than do blood neutrophils [5]. Here, we describe protocols to harvest mature murine bone marrow-derived neutrophils (BMDN) from mouse tibia and femur, and purify by discontinuous Percoll density gradient centrifugation [6]. BMDN collected from the 80/65 % Percoll interface contain >85 % BMDN, as confirmed by FACS analysis using antibodies against

Irving C. Allen (ed.), *Mouse Models of Innate Immunity: Methods and Protocols*, Methods in Molecular Biology, vol. 1031, DOI 10.1007/978-1-62703-481-4_5, © Springer Science+Business Media, LLC 2013

GR-1. To quantify NETs, BMDN are incubated with Sytox Green, a cell-impermeable fluorescent DNA dye. This ensures measurement of extracellular DNA from cells with compromised membrane integrity (typical during the formation of NETs), and not from viable, membrane-intact cells. Fluorescence emission is monitored following a 3-h incubation with the potent NET inducer phorbol 12-myristate 13-acetate (PMA) [7]. The percentage of NET formation can then be determined by subtracting the background fluorescence (determined with the addition of DNase), and dividing by the maximal fluorescence signal detected from lysed BMDN (during incubation with the detergent Triton X-100). NETs can also be visualized directly by first plating BMDN onto poly-L-lysine-coated coverslips, and then staining the fixed cells (resting or activated) with antibodies for the NET components histone H3 [7] or elastase [8], as well as DNA. Together, the protocols described are a complementary approach to quantify and visualize NETs.

2 Materials

2.1 Bone Marrow Neutrophil Isolation

1. 8–9-Week-old male or female C57BL/6 mice.
2. Laminar flow hood.
3. Small dissection scissors.
4. Forceps.
5. Lint-free wipes.
6. Sterile polyethylene disposable transfer pipettes.
7. 60 × 15 mm sterile polystyrene petri dishes.
8. 50 mL conical tubes.
9. 15 mL conical tubes.
10. 10 mL syringes.
11. $25G^{5/8}$ needles.
12. 20G needles.
13. 70 % ethanol.
14. Ice-cold deionized water.
15. Ice, ice-bucket.
16. MEM alpha cell culture medium 1× (Gibco). Store at 4 °C.
17. Phosphate-buffered saline (PBS) 1×, pH 7.4 without calcium chloride/magnesium chloride. Store at 4 °C.
18. Hank's Balanced Saline Solution (HBSS) with calcium chloride/magnesium chloride. Store at 4 °C.
19. Percoll density gradients: Prepare 100 % Percoll stock by mixing 90 mL of Percoll (pH 8.5–8.9) with 10 mL of 10× Dulbecco's phosphate-buffered saline. In a 50 mL conical

tube, prepare 80 % (mix 40 mL of 100 % Percoll with 10 mL of 1× PBS), 65 % (mix 32.5 mL of 100 % Percoll with 17.5 mL of 1× PBS), and 55 % (mix 27.5 mL of 100 % Percoll with 22.5 mL of 1× PBS) Percoll gradient solutions. Store at 4 °C.

20. 3.6 % (w/v) NaCl: Dissolve 3.6 g of NaCl in deionized water. Store at 4 °C.
21. Turk's solution: Dissolve 0.1 % crystal violet in 3 % acetic acid (prepared in sterile water). Shake vigorously. Store at room temperature.

2.2 Quantification of Neutrophil Extracellular DNA

1. BMDN (1×10^6 cells/mL).
2. Fluorescence microplate reader equipped with filters to detect excitation/emission maxima: 485/520 nm.
3. Humidified CO_2 incubator.
4. Black 96-well microplate.
5. 96-well microplate lids.
6. Microplate-sealing tape.
7. HBSS with calcium chloride/magnesium chloride. Store at 4 °C.
8. Sytox Green nucleic acid stain, 5 mM stock (Invitrogen). Protect from light and store at −20 °C. Just prior to addition to wells, prepare a 10× working solution (50 μM) by diluting 5 mM stock solution 1:100 with HBSS, into a foil-wrapped conical tube.
9. DNase 1 (RNase-free), 2 Units/μL. Store at −20 °C.
10. PMA, 1 mM stock (dissolve 1 mg of PMA in 1.62 mL dimethyl sulfoxide). Aliquot and store at −20 °C.
11. 10 % Triton X-100 (stock).

2.3 Immunofluorescence Visualization of NETs

1. BMDN (1×10^6 cells/mL).
2. Epi-fluorescence or confocal microscope equipped with filters to detect excitation/emission maxima: 358/461 nm (DAPI), 550/570 nm (TRITC), 495/519 nm (Alexa Fluor 488).
3. Humidified CO_2 incubator.
4. Sterile 12-well cell culture plates. Store at room temperature.
5. 12 mm round poly-L-lysine-coated glass coverslips. Store at 4 °C.
6. 75 × 25 × 1 mm microscope slides. Store at room temperature.
7. 1 mL microcentrifuge tubes.
8. Ice-cold methanol. Store at −20 °C.
9. PBS 1×, pH 7.4. Store at 4 °C.
10. PBS supplemented with Tween-20 (PBS-Tween). Mix 1 L PBS with 0.5 mL Tween-20. Store at room temperature.
11. 1 mM PMA stock. Dissolve 1 mg of PMA in 1.62 mL of dimethyl sulfoxide. Aliquot and store at −20 °C. Just prior to

use, prepare a 1 μM working stock solution by diluting 1:1,000-fold into HBSS. Store on ice until ready for use.

12. Fluorescent mounting medium. Store at 4 °C.
13. 4′,6-Diamidino-2-phenylindole, diacetate (DAPI; Invitrogen). Prepare a 5 mg/mL stock by dissolving 10 mg in 2 mL of deionized water. Solution may take some time to dissolve completely and may require sonication. For long-term storage, aliquot and store at −20 °C. For short-term storage store at 4 °C (stable for at least 6 months).
14. Histone H3 (D1H2) XP Rabbit monoclonal antibody (Cell Signaling). Store at −20 °C.
15. Neutrophil elastase polyclonal antibody (Abcam). Aliquot and store at -20 °C.
16. Goat anti-rabbit TRITC secondary antibody (Abcam). Aliquot and store at −20 °C.
17. Goat anti-rabbit Alexa Fluor 488 secondary antibody (Invitrogen). Store at 4 °C.
18. Blocking buffer: 3 % bovine serum albumin (BSA) prepared in PBS. Dissolve 0.3 g BSA in 10 mL of PBS. Store at 4 °C.

3 Methods

3.1 Bone Marrow-Derived Neutrophil Isolation

1. Sacrifice mouse by cervical dislocation (alternate methods such as CO_2 asphyxiation may also be utilized—refer to institutional guidelines).
2. In a laminar flow hood, spray the front (ventral) side of the mouse with 70 % ethanol, and make a lateral incision at the midline. Strip away the fur to expose the lower abdomen, soft tissue, and bone of the hind limbs (*see* **Note 1**).
3. Use scissors to make a cut above the hip joint, detach, and transfer intact hind limb to a 50 mL conical tube containing 20 mL of MEM alpha medium. Repeat with the second hind limb.
4. Gently cut away and remove soft tissue from the tibia and femur using scissors and lint-free wipes (*see* **Note 2**). Separate the tibia from the femur and transfer to a 60×15 mm petri dish containing MEM alpha medium. Repeat with the second hind limb.
5. Transfer tibias and femurs to a second petri dish containing 70 % ethanol. Soak the bones for ~30 s and then allow them to dry.
6. Use scissors to cut the proximal and distal ends off the tibia/femur, and flush the marrow into a third petri dish using a 10 mL syringe (containing 8 mL of MEM alpha medium) with a $25G^{5/8}$ needle attached (*see* **Note 3**).

7. Using a fresh syringe, attach a 20G needle and very gently aspirate the bone marrow to separate any clumps. This process should be repeated approximately four to five times. Repeat this procedure with the remaining bones.
8. Transfer to a 15 mL conical tube and centrifuge at 400 × *g* for 10 min at room temperature.
9. Gently pour off the supernatant and resuspend the cell pellet with 1 mL of PBS (without calcium chloride/magnesium chloride).
10. Prepare a Percoll density gradient. In a 15 mL conical tube, carefully add 4 mL of 80 % Percoll. Gently overlay this first layer with 3 mL of 65 % Percoll, followed by 3 mL of 55 % Percoll. Care should be taken to avoid mixing or disturbing the gradient solutions as they are added to the tube (*see* **Note 4**). Allow the Percoll tubes to stand for 5 min and then carefully add the cell suspension, prepared in **step 9**, to the top of the density gradient. Centrifuge at 1,000 × *g* for 30 min at room temperature, without braking.
11. Remove the centrifuge tube and visually inspect the gradient. The bone marrow neutrophils will have separated into the 80 %/65 % Percoll interface.
12. Gently dispose of the uppermost serum and 55 % Percoll layers using a disposable sterile transfer pipette. In a fresh 15 mL conical tube, collect the upper portion of the 65 % Percoll gradient and cells at the 80 %/65 % gradient interface. Top up volume to 14 mL with 1× PBS (without calcium chloride/magnesium chloride) and centrifuge at 400 × *g* for 10 min at 4 °C.
13. Pour off the supernatant and lyse the remaining red blood cells by gently resuspending the cell pellet in 3 mL of ice-cold deionized water. Leave undisturbed for 30 s. Add 1 mL of 3.6 % NaCl and mix gently. Centrifuge at 400 × *g* for 5 min at 4 °C.
14. Pour off the supernatant and gently resuspend the bone marrow-derived neutrophil cell pellet with 1 mL of HBSS (with calcium chloride/magnesium chloride). Determine the concentration using a neubauer hemocytometer. Mix 10 μL of cell suspension with 90 μL of HBSS and 5 μL of Turk's solution. Load 10 μL onto a hemocytometer.
15. Dilute bone marrow neutrophils to a concentration of 1×10^6 cells/mL using HBSS. Typically, ~6×10^6 bone marrow-derived neutrophils can be harvested per mouse.

3.2 Quantification of Extracellular DNA

The following protocol outlines the procedures for measuring neutrophil extracellular DNA, an index for the formation of NETs. BMDN (isolated in Subheading 3.1) or neutrophils from other

Table 1
Treatment conditions used for the quantification of neutrophil extracellular DNA (NETs)

	HBSS (μL)	BMDN (μL) (1×10^6/μL)	Triton X-100 (μL) (10 %)	PMA (μL) (1 μM)	DNase (μL) (2 U/μL)	Sytox green (μL) (50 μM)
BMDN	170	100	–	–	–	30
BMDN + Triton X-100	160	100	10	–	–	30
BMDN + PMA (100 nM)	140	100	–	30	–	30
BMDN + PMA (100 nM) + DNase	137.5	100	–	30	2.5	30
BMDN + DNase	167.5	100	–	–	2.5	30

sources (such as cell lines or peripheral blood) are plated at a density of 1×10^5 cells per well, and activated with PMA. The cell-impermeable DNA-binding dye, Sytox Green, is then added and the resulting fluorescence quantified on a fluorescence microplate reader. This protocol can be modified to incorporate other cell activators or additional inhibitors, and measurements made at variable time-points to monitor the kinetics of NET formation.

1. In a black 96-well microplate (*see* **Note 5**), prepare duplicates of the treatment wells shown in Table 1.
2. Using a pipette, add HBSS, 1×10^5 BMDN, and Triton X-100 (to determine total DNA content) or PMA (an activator of NET formation), as appropriate. Cover the microplate with a lid, and transfer to a humidified incubator (37 °C, 5 % CO_2).
3. After 2 h, add DNase to appropriate wells, and transfer back to the humidified incubator (37 °C, 5 % CO_2) (*see* **Note 6**).
4. After a further 45 min, carefully add 30 μL of SYTOX Green (10× working stock; 50 μM) to each well, mix, and transfer back to the humidified incubator. Allow to stand for a further 15 min, after which the plate can be sealed with microplate-sealing tape, and fluorescence quantified on a fluorescence microplate reader (*see* **Note 7**).
5. To quantify the amount of extracellular DNA (as a percentage of total DNA), subtract the fluorescence intensity of the DNase-containing wells from the comparative control, and divide by the fluorescence intensity emitted from "BMDN + Triton X-100" wells (total DNA present).

   Example:

$$\begin{array}{c}\text{Percentage total DNA} \\ \text{(induced by PMA)}\end{array} = \frac{\begin{array}{c}\text{Fluorescence Intensity}(\text{BMDN} + \text{PMA}) \\ -\text{Fluorescence Intensity}(\text{BMDN} + \text{PMA} + \text{DNase})\end{array}}{\text{Fluorescence Intensity}(\text{BMDN} + \text{Triton X} - 100)}$$

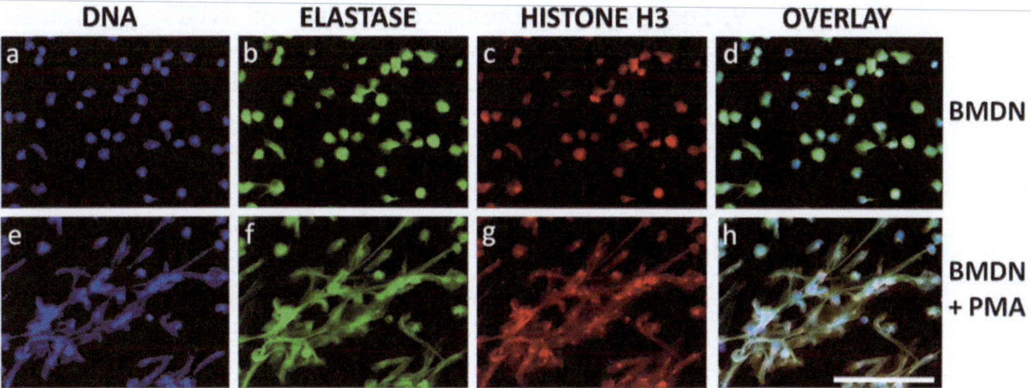

Fig. 1 Visualization of murine bone marrow-derived NETs by immunofluorescence microscopy. Resting BMDN or BMDN activated with PMA (100 μM, 3 h at 37 °C) were fixed and immunostained for DNA (DAPI; panels **a**, **e**), elastase (panels **b**, **f**), or histone H3 (panels **c**, **g**). Overlay of the three channels is shown in *panels* (**d**) and (**h**) for resting and PMA-activated BMDN, respectively. Scale bar = 100 μm

3.3 Immunofluorescence Visualization of NETs (See Fig. 1)

Visualization of NETs by immunofluorescence offers a complementary measure of extracellular DNA quantification, described in Subheading 3.2. While there are many markers for NETs, this protocol uses DAPI (to stain for DNA), as well as histone H3 and the serine protease elastase to label bone marrow NETs.

1. Place one poly-L-lysine-coated glass coverslip into each well of a sterile 12-well cell culture plate (*see* **Note 8**).
2. Plate BMDN onto the center of the poly-L-lysine-coated coverslips at a density of 1×10^5 cells, by gently pipetting 100 μL of BMDN cell suspension (1×10^6 cells/mL). To induce NETs with PMA (100 nM), mix 100 μL of BMDN cell suspension (1×10^6 cells/mL) with 15 μL of 10× PMA working stock solution (1 μM) and 35 μL of HBSS, in a separate microcentrifuge tube, before plating onto poly-L-lysine-coated coverslips. Replace the lid of the cell culture plate, and transfer to a humidified incubator (37 °C, 5 % CO_2) (*see* **Note 9**).
3. Incubate for 3 h.
4. Gently wash away cells that have not adhered with PBS. Aspirate with a pipette tip, and discard (*see* **Note 10**).
5. Transfer the cell culture plate, containing coverslips, to a fume hood and fix adherent cells by adding 400 μL of neutral-buffered formalin. Allow to stand for 15 min at room temperature.
6. Gently aspirate neutral-buffered formalin using a pipette tip, discard, and replace wells with 800 μL of PBS.
7. Repeat a further three times.
8. Transfer coverslips containing adherent BMDN to a new cell culture plate, containing 800 μL of PBS per well. Store at 4 °C (overnight) until ready to perform immunofluorescence labeling.

9. For immunofluorescence labeling of NETs, permeabilize adherent cells by transferring the prepared coverslips to a new cell culture plate, and add enough ice-cold 100 % methanol to sufficiently cover the surface (to a depth of 3.5 mm, ensuring that the cells do not dry out). Transfer to a –20 °C freezer and incubate for 10 min.
10. Aspirate with a pipette tip, and gently wash coverslips with PBS for 5 min.
11. Block nonspecific binding sites with blocking buffer (3 % BSA prepared in PBS) for 1 h at room temperature (*see* **Note 11**).
12. Aspirate with a pipette tip, and gently wash coverslips with PBS for 5 min.
13. To stain for histone H3, prepare primary histone H3 antibody (1:200 dilution) in blocking buffer supplemented with 0.3 % Triton X-100. Allow for 200 μL of diluted primary antibody per coverslip. For example, for 1 mL of diluted primary antibody, mix the following: 5 μL of histone H3 antibody, 33 μL of 10 % Triton X-100 (prepared with deionized water), and 962 μL of blocking buffer (3 % BSA prepared in PBS).
14. Transfer coverslips to a humidified chamber and incubate at 4 °C overnight, with gentle rotation (*see* **Note 12**).
15. Aspirate with a pipette tip, and gently wash coverslips with PBS-Tween for 5 min. Repeat three times.
16. Prepare goat anti-rabbit TRITC secondary antibody (1:400 dilution) in blocking buffer supplemented with 0.3 % Triton X-100. Pipette diluted antibody onto coverslips and incubate in a humidified chamber (protected from light) for 1 h at room temperature. For all subsequent steps, protect coverslips from light.
17. Aspirate with a pipette tip, and gently wash coverslips with PBS-Tween for 10 min. Repeat three times.
18. Incubate coverslips with blocking buffer (3 % BSA prepared in PBS) for 1 h at room temperature.
19. To stain for elastase, prepare primary elastase antibody (1:200 dilution) in blocking buffer supplemented with 0.3 % Triton X-100. Pipette diluted antibody onto coverslips, and incubate in a humidified chamber (protected from light) for 1 h at room temperature.
20. Aspirate with a pipette tip, and gently wash coverslips with PBS-Tween for 5 min. Repeat three times.
21. Prepare goat anti-rabbit Alexa Fluor 488 secondary antibody (1:400 dilution) in blocking buffer supplemented with 0.3 % Triton X-100. Transfer coverslips to a humidified chamber (protected from light), and incubate for 1 h at room temperature.

22. Aspirate with a pipette tip, and gently wash coverslips with PBS-Tween for 10 min. Repeat three times.
23. To counterstain for DNA, incubate coverslips with 1:12,500 dilution of DAPI (mix 0.4 μL of DAPI stock solution with 5 mL of PBS), for 5 min at room temperature.
24. Aspirate with a pipette tip, and gently wash coverslips with PBS. Repeat several times.
25. Mount coverslips using a small drop of fluorescent mounting medium per microscope slide (*see* **Note 13**). Allow the preparation to dry overnight by storing the slides in a slide holder at room temperature, protected from light. Thereafter, transfer to 4 °C for storage.
26. Visualize the DNA, histone H3, and elastase staining on a confocal or epi-fluorescence microscope, equipped with filters suitable for DAPI (excitation/emission: 358/461 nm), TRITC (excitation/emission: 550/570 nm), and Alexa Fluor 488 (excitation/emission: 495/519 nm).

4 Notes

1. Spraying with ethanol helps to reduce the amount of fur that sticks to exposed tissue. Make a shallow cut or incision with scissors so as to not pierce the intestinal tract, and continue cutting laterally to completely remove skin from the lower abdomen to hind paws.
2. Hold the tibia/femur between your thumb and forefinger, and use lint-free wipes (providing more friction) to remove the surrounding soft tissue.
3. Flush the bone marrow out, using about 2 mL of media per tibia/femur. The bones should appear transparent afterwards.
4. Percoll gradients should be slowly added to the conical tube, with the tip of disposable transfer pipette touching the tube wall. If added too quickly, the separation of bone marrow cells between the discontinuous gradients will be less effective.
5. Black microplates are used for fluorescence assays as they reduce the level of autofluorescence and therefore background signal.
6. DNase can be added to the assay 60 min before quantification of extracellular DNA. If increasing or reducing the overall incubation period (i.e., from 3 h), adjust accordingly.
7. Sytox green is added to the assay 15 min before the quantification of extracellular DNA. If increasing or reducing the overall incubation period (i.e., from 3 h), adjust the timepoint at which the DNA stain is added accordingly. Prior to measurement,

briefly shake the plate to mix the well contents. This option is available on most microplate readers.

8. 12-Well cell culture plates are used to contain the coverslips, although other holders such as petri dishes can also be used. Ensure that, if using 24-well plates, the coverslips can be removed with forceps without breaking.
9. At least 2–3 replicates of each treatment should be prepared, as the cell suspension occasionally leaks from the coverslip (onto the cell culture plate surface), and can then no longer be used.
10. NETs are very fragile and can easily be dislodged. Sufficient care should be taken during all washes. Only use a pipette, and gently aspirate.
11. Blocking buffer can be prepared the day before, and stored at 4 °C for at least a week.
12. An easy alternative to commercially available but expensive chambers is to line a shallow plastic container (large enough to hold the tissue culture plate, containing coverslips) with moistened paper towels, and replace the lid.
13. To mount the coverslips, place a small drop of fluorescent mounting medium onto the surface of a glass microscope slide. Use forceps to pick up the coverslip, and gently dry the underside on paper towel or lint-free wipes. Place one edge of the coverslip just outside of the mounting medium, and lower until it comes into contact with the medium. Release the remainder of the coverslip to allow the mounting medium to distribute evenly.

References

1. Borregaard N (2010) Neutrophils, from marrow to microbes. Immunity 33:657–670
2. Brinkmann V, Reichard U, Goosmann C, Fauler B, Uhlemann Y, Weiss DS, Weinrauch Y, Zychlinsky A (2004) Neutrophil extracellular traps kill bacteria. Science 303:1532–1535
3. Papayannopoulos V, Metzler K, Hakkim A, Zychlinksky A (2010) Neutrophil elastase and myeloperoxidase regulate the formation of neutrophil extracellular traps. J Cell Biol 191: 677–691
4. Urban C, Ermert D, Schmid M, Abu-Abed U, Goosmann C, Nacken W, Brinkmann V, Jungblut PR, Zychlinsky A (2009) Neutrophil extracellular traps contain calprotectin, a cytosolic protein complex involved in host defense against Candida albicans. PLoS Pathog 5:e1000639
5. Boxio R, Bossenmeyer-Pourie C, Steinckwich N, Dournon C, Nusse O (2004) Mouse bone marrow contains large numbers of functionally competent neutrophils. J Leukoc Biol 75:604–611
6. Chervenick PA, Boggs DR, Marsh JC, Cartwright GE, Wintrobe MM (1968) Quantitative studies of blood and bone marrow neutrophils in normal mice. Am J Physiol 215:353–360
7. Fuchs TA, Abed C, Goosmann R, Hurwitz R, Schulze I, Wahn V, Weinrauch Y, Brinkmann V, Zychlinsky A (2007) Novel cell death program leads to neutrophil extracellular traps. J Cell Biol 176:231–241
8. Lim MB, Kuiper JW, Katchky A, Goldberg H, Glogauer M (2011) Rac2 is required for the formation of neutrophil extracellular traps. J Leukoc Biol 90:771–776

Chapter 6

Assessment of Oxidative Metabolism

Emilie Imbeault and Denis Gris

Abstract

Oxidative metabolism is one of the central physiological processes that regulate multiple functions in a cell including cell death and survival, proliferation, gene transcription, and protein modification. There are multitudes of techniques that are used to evaluate oxidative activity. Here, we summarize how to measure oxidative activity by flow cytometry. This versatile technique allows the evaluation of the level of oxidative activity within heterogeneous populations of cells and in cell culture. Flow cytometry is a quick method that yields highly reproducible results with small sample volumes. Therefore, it is an ideal technique for evaluating changes in oxidative activity in samples from mice.

Key words Oxidative metabolism, Oxidative activity, Flow cytometry, Fluorescent dyes, Whole blood, Cell culture

1 Introduction

The evaluation of oxidative metabolism efficiency is a useful measure of physiological activity in the cell. The oxidative state of a cell regulates fundamental processes of cell metabolism including proliferation, survival, inflammation, DNA damage/repair, and cell death. Not surprisingly, many diseases are associated with defects in the regulation of oxidative metabolism, which include neurodegeneration, carcinogenesis, diabetes, and atherosclerosis [1]. For example, mutation of the gene encoding the SOD protein results in increased oxidation in motor neurons and leads to amyotrophic lateral sclerosis (ALS)-like pathology. On the other hand, a defect in neutrophil-associated NADPH oxidase, which leads to deficiency in the production of superoxide and hydrogen peroxide, is an underlying mechanism of chronic granulomatosis disease. Oxidative activity can be described as a sum concentration of oxidative reagents in the cell at any given time. Most prominent contributors of oxidative activity are reactive nitrogen species (RNS) and reactive oxygen species (ROS). ROS consists of

Irving C. Allen (ed.), *Mouse Models of Innate Immunity: Methods and Protocols*, Methods in Molecular Biology, vol. 1031, DOI 10.1007/978-1-62703-481-4_6, © Springer Science+Business Media, LLC 2013

hydrogen peroxide (H_2O_2) and substances containing unpaired electrons, which include superoxide, peroxyl, and hydroperoxyl.

The generation of ROS is dependent on NADPH oxidases, which consists of multiple members of the *NOX* gene family (Nox1-5). RNS comprise peroxynitrites (ONOO–), which are downstream of nitric oxide syntheses. The level of oxidative activity can be measured by the amount of damaged cell material, such as DNA, RNA, protein, and lipids [2–4]. Increased oxidative activity is counterbalanced by increased expression of the reducing enzymes that protect cells from the harmful environment of reactive oxygen and nitrogen species. Therefore, another way to measure oxidative activity is to measure the expression of antioxidants that accumulate in a cell in response to the presence of ROS and RNS [5].

Several methods that measure oxidative activity have been developed. For example, the nitrobluetetrazolium precipitation reduction test is a crude method that evaluates high levels of oxidative activity and it requires large sample volumes [6]. Likewise, chemiluminescence is a highly sensitive and easily quantified method that can be used with small 20–100 μl sample sizes [7]. Chemiluminescence can measure the level of oxidative activity in a homogeneous cell population [8]. Lastly, flow cytometry is a very sensitive way to evaluate oxidative activity in heterogeneous cell populations, as well as in homogeneous cell populations. This review describes one of the ways that flow cytometry can be utilized to measure the oxidative activity of a cell.

Several detection dyes have been developed that are useful to measure oxidative activity by flow cytometry. Upon oxidation, dyes such as 2′7′-dichlorofluorescein (DCFH), DCFH diacetate (DCFH-DA), and dihydrorhodamine 123 (DHR) fluoresce when excited with a 488 nm laser. From our experience, DHR 123 typically yields the most accurate and reproducible results. In addition, DHR easily penetrates into live cells *in vivo* and can be used to evaluate the oxidative state within tissues using microscopy, fluorometry, and flow cytometry. For this reason, this review concentrates on the protocols using DHR to measure oxidative activity using flow cytometry. This assay can be used to quantify the oxidative activity of cells in whole blood, bone marrow, spleen, and other tissues. Also, we and others have successfully utilized this technique to measure the oxidative activity of THP-1 monocytic cell lines, RAW mouse monocytic cell lines, primary mouse astrocytes, and mouse embryonic fibroblasts [9–11].

2 Materials

1. Mouse blood sample, primary cells, or cell line: This procedure has been successfully performed using human and rodent blood samples and multiple human and mouse cell lines. At least 100 μl

of whole blood is required to measure the oxidative activity of neutrophils, monocytes, T cells, and B cells. For mouse primary cells and cell lines, $0.5–1 \times 10^7$ cells are required.

2. RPMI-1640.
3. 12×75 mm test tubes.
4. Heparinized syringes.
5. Cell culture centrifuge capable to spin at 300×*g*.
6. Water bath 37 °C.
7. Liquid nitrogen.
8. Flow cytometer equipped with an argon laser and a photomultiplier tube (PMT) with a 525 nm band-pass filter.
9. 10× Lysis buffer: 82.5 g of ammonium chloride (NH_4Cl), 10 g of potassium bicarbonate ($KHCO_3$), 0.37 g of ethylenediaminetetraacetic acid (EDTA), and bring the volume up to 1 l using ddH_2O (*see* **Note 1**).
10. Prepare 4 % formaldehyde from powder. To completely dissolve paraformaldehyde heat the solution to 60 °C on a stir plate. Several drops of NaOH may help to clear the solution.
11. Fixation buffer: 1.7 % formaldehyde and 2 % fetal bovine serum (FBS) in phosphate-buffered saline (PBS) (*see* **Note 2**).
12. Dihydrorhodamine 123 (DHR) (Sigma): Add 2.5 mg/ml of DHR in DMSO for the stoke concentration and divide this stock into small aliquots of 30–50 μl. Store the aliquots in liquid nitrogen (*see* **Note 3**). Before an experiment, prepare a 1/1,000 working solution (2.5 μg/ml) in RPMI 1640. Prepare 100 μl of working DHR solution for each 400 μl sample.
13. Phorbol 12-myristate 13-acetate (PMA) (Sigma): Dissolve 1 mg/ml of PMA in DMSO and divide this stock solution into small aliquots of 30–50 μl. Freeze each aliquot at −80 °C. Prepare a 1/100 working solution and prepare to use 5 μl per sample.

3 Methods

1. Prepare DHR, PMA, and any experimental reagents for cell stimulation (such as pathogen-associated molecular pattern (PAMP) molecules or damage-associated molecular patterns (DAMPs)) to specified concentrations in separate tubes (12×75 mm test tubes). Each tube should contain 300 μl of RPMI 1640 and 100 μl of DHR (*see* **Note 4**). The tubes should be labeled as follows: Tube #1 "Cells only," which will contain 100 μl of RPMI 1640 instead of DHR; Tube #2 "Cells DHR ice"; Tube #3 "Cells DHR"; Tube #4 "Cells DHR+PMA"; Tube #5 "Cells DHR + reagent of interest." The concentration

of each reagent of interest should enable 5 μl of the reagent to be added to each sample (*see* **Note 5**).

2. Put the "DHR ice" tubes on ice; the rest of the tubes can be placed at 37 °C (*see* **Note 6**).
3. Collect blood from experimental mice by heart stick into a heparinized syringe and aliquot 100 μl into each of the test tubes. Make sure to thoroughly resuspend the samples (*see* **Note 7**). Incubate each sample for 15 min at 37 °C.
4. Spin cells for 5 min at 280 × *g*. Resuspend the cell pellet in 1 ml of lysis buffer and incubate for 5 min at room temperature (*see* **Note 8**). Following the incubation, add 3 ml of ice-cold PBS.
5. Centrifuge the cells at 4 °C for 5 min at 280 × *g* and resuspend the cells in fixative buffer. If any surface staining is desired then cells should be re-suspended in blocking buffer (*see* **Note 9**).
6. Surface staining is performed according to routine protocols (*see* **Note 10**).
7. Scan cells using a flow cytometer (Fig. 1) (*see* **Note 11**).
8. Cells incubated on ice with DHR may have high levels of nonphysiologically relevant background staining. Therefore, special care must be taken to use quiescent cells. Incubation with PMA shows the oxidative capacity of cells. The concentration of PMA used in this protocol will push cells to the near-maximum oxidative activity, which is also referred to as an oxidative burst, while staining with DHR only gives an idea of the level of oxidative activity at rest.
9. The intense brightness of the staining with DHR123 usually results in a skewed readout of the population of cells (Fig. 1b). Therefore, the geometrical mean florescence intensity should be used for analysis rather than mean florescence intensity.
10. In the case when several peaks of fluorescence (Fig. 1c) can be distinguished within one population, this population can be separated into "high" and "low" populations. When working with small changes (Fig. 1d), the percent of positive cells in the specifically assigned gate might be a more useful measure than the geometrical mean of fluorescent intensity.
11. Data should be analyzed using a multiple comparison test (*see* **Notes 12**).

4 Notes

1. This 10× formulation is stable at room temperature for at least 6 months. Prepare fresh 1× buffer before each experiment.
2. The concentration of 1.7 % was determined to be the optimal concentration of fixative for intracellular and surface staining [12].

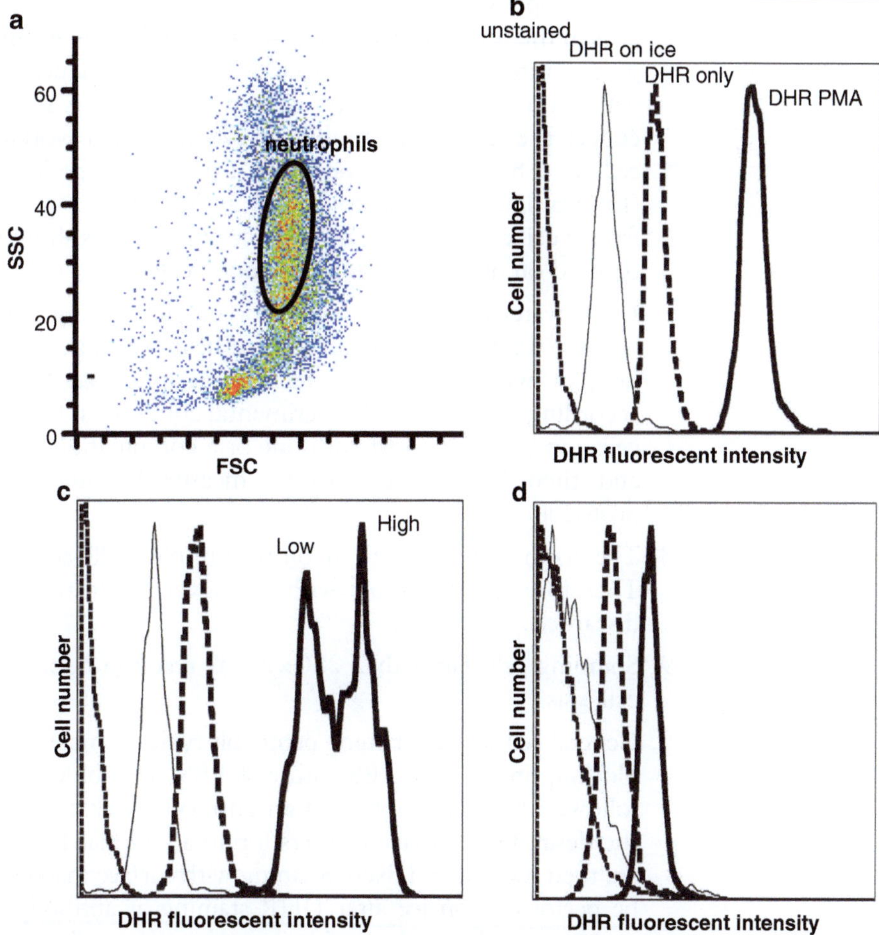

Fig. 1 Examples of data. (**a**) Side scatter and forward scatter of mouse blood sample. (**b**), (**c**), and (**d**) overlay histograms of 4 samples (the *thin dashed line* represents unstained cells; the *thin line* represents DHR on ice; the *thick dashed line* represents DHR only; and the *thick line* represents DHR + PMA) of (**b**) neutrophils from gate, (**c**) neutrophils from a different experiment, and (**d**) human THP1 cells

3. DHR 123 is easily oxidized. Storage in liquid nitrogen minimizes batch-to-batch variation over time. Once the aliquot of DHR123 has been thawed, it can be stored at −20 °C for several weeks with repeated freeze–thaw cycles.

4. It is very important to use the same batch of regents within the same series of experiments in order to increase the reproducibility of the data.

5. The negative control cells (cells incubated on ice–ice negative control), the DHR-only-treated cells, and the positive control PMA-stimulated cells are all required conditions for each experiment that may reveal mishandling of cells during the procedure. Also, these conditions allow the user to identify the relative oxidative activity of a cell compared to its oxidative potential.

6. The sample size can be reduced depending on the amount of cells in the population of interest. At least 10,000 events in the gate of interest must be collected. In our experience, working with mouse neutrophils, 50 μl of whole blood is sufficient to collect the necessary number of events. When working with cells that have been activated for a prolonged period of time (for example, blood samples after an infection or primed cells from a cell culture) the DHR on ice control cells should always be used on nonactivated/non-primed cells.
7. Use a water bath rather than a forced air exchange incubator because water has a superior level of heat exchange. Gently mix samples every 5 min. The incubation time may be adjusted according to the desired experimental conditions. For example, cells can be primed first with one or a combination of reagents and then fluorescence can be measured using the above protocol.
8. The formation of clots in blood samples will activate cells. Therefore, every sample with any level of clotting must be discarded.
9. Spinning cells faster than $280 \times g$ may result in poor red blood cell lysis.
10. General cell surface staining protocols typically include 5 min of blocking in 30 μl of PBS with 5 % FBS. This blocking is then followed by incubation with an antibody cocktail specific for the desired cell surface markers for an additional 15 min. Cells are then washed and fixed. Staining with surface markers should be performed on ice after DHR staining as antibody binding may change the level of oxidative activity in a cell. In this case, cells should be fixed after surface staining is complete.
11. Ideally, samples should be analyzed by the flow cytometer immediately after staining. This will allow the fixation step to be skipped. However, when working with human samples, the fixation step is required. In addition, fixing cells allows samples to be scanned within 24 or even 48 h.
12. Usually in each experiment, an n of at least 4 should be performed. This should be followed by an ANOVA statistical analysis. A *t*-test is not suitable since more than two conditions are compared with each experiment.

References

1. Ray PD, Huang BW, Tsuji Y (2012) Reactive oxygen species (ROS) homeostasis and redox regulation in cellular signaling. Cell Signal 24(5):981–990
2. Shacter E (2000) Quantification and significance of protein oxidation in biological samples. Drug Metab Rev 32(3–4):307–326
3. Halliwell B, Dizdaroglu M (1992) The measurement of oxidative damage to DNA by HPLC and GC/MS techniques. Free Radic Res Comm 16(2):75–87
4. Moore K, Roberts LJ 2nd (1998) Measurement of lipid peroxidation. Free Radic Res 28(6): 659–671

5. Vives-Bauza C, Starkov A, Garcia-Arumi E (2007) Measurements of the antioxidant enzyme activities of superoxide dismutase, catalase, and glutathione peroxidase. Meth Cell Biol 80:379–393
6. Bellinati-Pires R, Waitzberg DL, Salgado MM, Carneiro-Sampaio MM (1993) Functional alterations of human neutrophils by medium-chain triglyceride emulsions: evaluation of phagocytosis, bacterial killing, and oxidative activity. J Leukoc Biol 53(4):404–410
7. Dahlgren C, Karlsson A (1999) Respiratory burst in human neutrophils. J Immunol Meth 232(1–2):3–14
8. Vladimirov YA, Proskurnina EV (2009) Free radicals and cell chemiluminescence. Biochem Biokhimiia 74(13):1545–1566
9. Gris D, Hamilton EF, Weaver LC (2008) The systemic inflammatory response after spinal cord injury damages lungs and kidneys. Exp Neurol 211(1):259–270
10. Allen IC, Moore CB, Schneider M, Lei Y, Davis BK, Scull MA et al (2011) NLRX1 protein attenuates inflammatory responses to infection by interfering with the RIG-I-MAVS and TRAF6-NF-kappaB signaling pathways. Immunity 34(6):854–865
11. Farrell SM, Groeger G, Bhatt L, Finnegan S, O'Brien CJ, Cotter TG (2011) bFGF-mediated redox activation of the PI3K/Akt pathway in retinal photoreceptor cells. Eur J Neurosci 33(4):632–641
12. Krutzik PO, Nolan GP (2006) Fluorescent cell barcoding in flow cytometry allows high-throughput drug screening and signaling profiling. Nat Methods 3(5):361–368

Chapter 7

Generation and Culture of Mouse Embryonic Fibroblasts

Yu Lei

Abstract

The innate immune system is evolutionarily conserved and shared by a wide spectrum of cells, including epithelial cells, endothelial cells, fibroblasts, macrophages, dendritic cells, and lymphocytes. The extensive utilization of genetically manipulated animals in innate immunity studies has become the standard approach to confirm functional data acquired in cell lines. The easy generation and physiological relevance of mouse embryonic fibroblasts (MEFs) have made them a powerful tool in discovering novel signaling pathways, investigating regulatory networks, and exploring biochemical profiling of protein complexes involved in innate immune responses. Due to their extensive use, this chapter aims to provide a protocol for generating, maintaining, and storing primary MEFs for those who have minimal experience in animal models. Precautions and notes are integrated into the description of each step of the protocol for the benefits of minimizing unnecessary cross-referencing.

Key words Innate immunity, Mouse embryonic fibroblasts, MEF

1 Introduction

Recent advances in immunology have heavily relied on the generation and exploration of gene deletion or transgenic mouse models. The extensive utilization of these genetically manipulated animals has become the standard approach to confirm the functional data acquired in cell lines. Innate immunity studies witnessed exponential development in recent years thanks to the discoveries of novel families of pathogen-associated molecular pattern receptors, immune adaptor molecules, intricate regulatory networks of innate immune responses, and novel co-stimulatory/co-inhibitory pathways [1–3]. In contrast to the involvement of highly specialized antigen-presenting cells and lymphocytes in the adaptive immune system, innate immunity is an evolutionarily conserved system shared by a wide spectrum of cells, including but not limited to epithelial cells, endothelial cells, fibroblasts, macrophages, dendritic cells, and lymphocytes. Importantly, due to the anatomic

Irving C. Allen (ed.), *Mouse Models of Innate Immunity: Methods and Protocols*, Methods in Molecular Biology, vol. 1031, DOI 10.1007/978-1-62703-481-4_7,

features of mammalian tissues, epithelial cells and fibroblasts often constitute the primary physical barrier of the host against a variety of microbial or environmental insults. Hence, these cells are equipped with cytoplasmic sensors and the necessary innate immune signaling pathways to be readily engaged with host–pathogen interactions. Given the functional relevance and easy generation of mouse embryonic fibroblasts (MEFs), these cells are extensively used in biochemical identification and functional characterization of novel players in the innate immune system. In fact, some emerging families of these sensors are extensively studied in MEFs [4–9]. This chapter provides a standard protocol for the generation and culture of MEFs. Of special note, the protocol involving the generation and the use of MEFs must be reviewed and approved by the appropriate regulatory bodies at each institution (i.e., the Institutional Animal Care and Use Committee, IACUC). Likewise, the breeding and care for mice must also follow all official guidelines.

2 Materials

2.1 Mice

1. At least 2 breeding cages of mice for each genotype need to be tested. Each breeding cage should include 1 male and 2 female mice, 6–12 weeks of age (*see* **Note 1**).

2.2 Reagents

1. Phosphate-buffered saline (PBS 1×), pH 7.4.
2. Dulbecco's modified Eagle medium (DMEM).
3. Fetal bovine serum (FBS).
4. 100× Penicillin–streptomycin (10,000 units of penicillin and 10,000 μg of streptomycin/ml).
5. Trypsin–EDTA 0.25 % solution.
6. Freezing medium: 10 % Dimethyl sulfoxide (DMSO), 20 % FBS, 70 % DMEM high glucose, and 1 % penicillin–streptomycin (*see* **Note 2**).

2.3 Supplies and Equipment

1. Culture dishes and conical tubes: 60- and 100-mm tissue culture dishes; 15 and 50 ml conical tubes; and 2 ml screw cap cryovials.
2. Laminar flow hood (*see* **Note 3**).
3. Sterile 40 μm cell strainers.
4. Surgical instruments: Dissecting forceps, scissors, and razor/scalpel blades (*see* **Note 4**).

3 Methods

3.1 Establish Timed Breeding Cages (See Note 5)

1. Place 1 male mouse with 2 female mice.
2. Examine the female mice for the presence of copulation plugs each morning until the plug is identified.
3. Once the plug is identified, transfer the female mice to a new cage and note the time of embryo development as 0.5 days.
4. Allow the embryos to develop for 13.5–15.5 days. The most widely accepted ages for the embryos used in MEF generation are between 13.5 and 15.5 days.

3.2 Pre-surgical Preparations

1. Pregnant mice should be euthanized as specified in an approved animal protocol. The most widely used methods include the use of carbon dioxide, isoflurane overdose, or avertin overdose. The primary method should be followed by a secondary physical method, such as cervical dislocation.
2. Spray the entire mouse with 70 % ethanol.
3. The dissection should be performed in a laminar flow hood (*see* **Note 6**).
4. In a clean area under the hood, label PBS-filled 100-mm tissue culture plates with the genotype of each mouse and a unique number to identify each embryo (*see* **Note 7**).

3.3 Dissect the Embryos

1. Lift the abdominal wall with blunt forceps and make a shallow 3-mm transverse incision. Next, make a longitudinal incision to expose the abdominal wall. At this point, the uterus with embryos should be easily visible. Take all precautions to keep the surgical site uncontaminated. If the surgical instruments are contaminated by hair, fully rinse the instrument in 70 % ethanol or use a new set of instruments.
2. Expose the embryos by opening the abdominal wall. Take special precautions to avoid damaging the internal organs in the peritoneal cavity, especially the small intestine and colon. Damage to these organs increases the risk of contaminating the embryos with bacteria.
3. Carefully transfer each embryo, with intact yolk sac, to the tissue culture plates prepared in Subheading 3.2, **step 4**.

3.4 Prepare the Fetuses

1. Tease apart the yolk sac with a pair of fine forceps and discard the yolk sac.
2. Carefully remove the fetus head and keep it in a separate PBS-filled conical tube labeled with its genotype and identifying number. This identification should match the respective

100-mm tissue culture plate. The fetal remains that are not used for MEF generation, including the head, are used for genotyping.

3. Carefully remove and discard dark red internal organs, including heart, liver, and lung.
4. Wash each prepared fetus in PBS and transfer it to a new 60-mm tissue culture dish that has been identically labeled as the original plate.

3.5 Prepare the MEF Suspension

1. Add 3 ml of prechilled 0.25 % trypsin–EDTA to each dish.
2. Mince the fetus tissue thoroughly with two razor or scalpel blades. This step is critical for enhancing the final yield of MEFs. It is important that this step be thoroughly conducted and not rushed.
3. Gently pipet all of the tissue fragment suspensions up and down ten times.
4. Incubate each tissue culture dish at 37 °C for 10 min. Do not expose cells to extended trypsin treatment. Extensive exposure to trypsin will markedly reduce cell viability.
5. Transfer the suspension to a 40 μm cell strainer placed on a 50 ml conical tube and allow cell suspension to flow through the cell strainer with gravity.
6. Spin the cells down at 500 × *g* and 4 °C for 5 min. Wash the cell pellets once with prechilled complete DMEM medium containing 10 % FBS to deactivate and remove any residual trypsin.

3.6 Passage 0 MEF Culture

1. Cell pellets from the previous step are resuspended in complete culture media.
2. Add 11 ml of culture medium to each of the 100-mm culture dishes or 75-mm^2 culture flasks.
3. Culture the cells in a standard humidified 37 °C, 5 % CO_2 incubator for 24 h. If all of the previous steps are followed properly, the cells should be close to confluence. These cells are considered to be at passage 0 (*see* **Note 8**).

3.7 Harvest MEFs (See Note 9)

1. Following the initial passage, split cells when they reach approximately 70 % confluence.
2. Remove culture medium and gently wash cells two times with PBS.
3. Add 4 ml of 0.05 % trypsin–EDTA solution to the culture dish, and incubate at 37 °C for 3 min. Shake one to two times during the incubation.

4. Deactivate the trypsin and resuspend the cells with 15 ml complete culture medium. Spin down the cell pellets at $500 \times g$ and 4 °C for 5 min.
5. Wash the pellets one time with PBS and resuspend in 15 ml complete culture medium for passage.

3.8 Freeze and Thaw MEFs

1. Resuspend 1.0×10^6 MEFs in 1 ml of freezing medium, and transfer to a pre-labeled cryovial.
2. Place cryovials in the controlled rate freezer for 24 h and then transfer them to liquid nitrogen for long-term cryopreservation (*see* **Note 10**).
3. When thawing cells from frozen stocks, remove cells from liquid nitrogen and immediately place the cryovials in a 37 °C water bath.
4. Transfer the cell suspension to a 50 ml conical tube, and add pre-warmed complete culture media dropwise into the suspension. Then spin down the cells and proceed with Subheadings 3.6 and 3.7.

4 Notes

1. Although the use of wild-type mice from the same genetic background is commonly accepted as controls for MEF generation, we highly recommend generating littermate control cells for better accuracy. If gene manipulation does not result in breeding failure or death at early embryonic stages, then the use of heterozygous breeding pairs are recommended. The male-to-female mouse ratio should be 1:2 in the breeding cages.
2. Be very careful when handling DMSO, which is a known carcinogenic chemical and could penetrate intact skin.
3. We recommend using different hoods for generating MEFs and regular cell culture to minimize the chances of contamination.
4. All instruments should be sterilized by autoclaving prior to experiments.
5. Timed breeding is critical for the successful preparation of MEFs. The most widely used approach to determine the starting date of embryo development is the identification of a copulation plug (semen plug) in the vagina. Although it is usually identifiable before 8:00 a.m., it should be noted that the copulation plug can be hard to recognize 12 h after mating. In addition, it is more difficult to identify the plug in very young mice. Hence, copulation plugs need to be examined early in the morning every day until it is identified. The time when a copulation plug is identified will be marked as day 0.5

for embryo development. All female mice should then be transferred to a new cage for the next 13–15 days.

6. Due to the thick hair, it can be challenging to keep the dissection process sterile. Thus, it is of critical importance to take all available precautions to reduce the potential for contamination. It is advisable to separate relatively "clean areas" and relatively "dirty areas" in the hood after transferring mice into the working space. Embryo dissection should be confined to the "dirty area," and all subsequent procedures should be performed in the "clean area."
7. Clear numbering of the plates will greatly benefit subsequent genotyping and matching the results to each of the dissected embryos.
8. Primary MEFs maintain active proliferation for about 4 passages. The proliferation rates will considerably drop after 5 passages. Hence, only early-passage cells are appropriate for downstream applications. Active MEFs typically double in cell number every 48 h. Hence, it is recommended to freeze passages 0 and 1 MEFs for the convenience of further experimentation.
9. The culture and maintenance of MEFs are similar to other fibroblast cell lines.
10. There are a number of affordable controlled rate freezers available from different vendors. The principle is to decrease the ambient temperature gradually. Do not directly place cryovials into liquid nitrogen. This will significantly reduce cell viability.

References

1. Davis BK, Wen H, Ting JP (2011) The inflammasome NLRs in immunity, inflammation, and associated diseases. Annu Rev Immunol 29:707–735
2. Ting JP, Duncan JA, Lei Y (2010) How the noninflammasome NLRs function in the innate immune system. Science 327:286–290
3. Wen H, Lei Y, Eun SY, Ting JP (2010) Plexin-A4-semaphorin 3A signaling is required for Toll-like receptor- and sepsis-induced cytokine storm. J Exp Med 207:2943–2957
4. Ishikawa H, Barber GN (2008) STING is an endoplasmic reticulum adaptor that facilitates innate immune signalling. Nature 455: 674–678
5. Seth RB, Sun L, Ea CK, Chen ZJ (2005) Identification and characterization of MAVS, a mitochondrial antiviral signaling protein that activates NF-kappaB and IRF 3. Cell 122: 669–682
6. Yoneyama M, Kikuchi M, Natsukawa T, Shinobu N, Imaizumi T et al (2004) The RNA helicase RIG-I has an essential function in double-stranded RNA-induced innate antiviral responses. Nat Immunol 5:730–737
7. Kawai T, Takahashi K, Sato S, Coban C, Kumar H et al (2005) IPS-1, an adaptor triggering RIG-I- and Mda5-mediated type I interferon induction. Nat Immunol 6:981–988
8. Meylan E, Curran J, Hofmann K, Moradpour D, Binder M et al (2005) Cardif is an adaptor protein in the RIG-I antiviral pathway and is targeted by hepatitis C virus. Nature 437: 1167–1172
9. Allen IC, Moore CB, Schneider M, Lei Y, Davis BK et al (2011) NLRX1 protein attenuates inflammatory responses to infection by interfering with the RIG-I-MAVS and TRAF6-NF-kappaB signaling pathways. Immunity 34: 854–865

Chapter 8

Primary Ear Fibroblast Derivation from Mice

Chris B. Moore and Irving C. Allen

Abstract

Mouse embryonic fibroblasts (MEFs) are commonly utilized as a primary cell culture model and have several advantages over other types of ex vivo-derived cells. However, the successful generation of MEFs is time consuming and requires a certain level of mouse expertise to successfully complete. Thus, primary ear-derived fibroblasts offer an acceptable alternative to MEFs. Fibroblasts derived from the pinna of adult mice are easily attainable with minimal skill, proliferate rapidly, and are easy to manipulate. Likewise, because they are derived from adult mice, other organs can be concurrently harvested for the isolation of additional types of primary cells. Similar to MEFs, ear fibroblasts are an excellent ex vivo model system to study mechanisms associated with virus infection and produce a diverse array of inflammatory mediators, such as cytokines and interferon. Here, we describe a highly versatile and simple method for the derivation, maintenance, and viral challenge of primary ear-derived fibroblasts from mice.

Key words Fibroblast, Interferon, Vesicular stomatitis virus, VSV, Mouse embryonic fibroblast, MEF, Mouse primary cell, Innate immunity, Virus, Ex vivo

1 Introduction

Genetically modified mice are essential tools used to define the role of specific genes in the innate immune response to pathogens. While studies in whole animals provide critical insight into the physiological relevance of a particular gene, it is often necessary to limit the complexity of the model system in order to resolve key aspects of the underlying mechanism. This is typically accomplished through the use of ex vivo primary cells. Mouse embryonic fibroblasts (MEFs) are a commonly utilized and attractive ex vivo model system for a diverse range of applications associated with the host innate immune response. MEFs offer a well-characterized model that is amenable to challenge with a diverse range of viruses and bacteria. The cells are easy to manipulate and following stimulation, MEFs are robust producers of inflammatory mediators, such as type I interferons and cytokines. However, the generation of MEFs is a time-consuming endeavor and requires a high level of

Irving C. Allen (ed.), *Mouse Models of Innate Immunity: Methods and Protocols*, Methods in Molecular Biology, vol. 1031, DOI 10.1007/978-1-62703-481-4_8, © Springer Science+Business Media, LLC 2013

animal expertise to successfully time the pregnancies for optimal harvest. Thus, under certain experimental conditions or for laboratories with limited mouse expertise, it may be more appropriate to utilize primary ear fibroblasts harvested from adult mice as an alternative approach to MEFs. Primary ear fibroblasts have all of the advantages typically associated with MEFs, can be rapidly generated, and require very little mouse expertise to harvest. Likewise, it is also possible to harvest other tissues for primary cell derivation, such as bone marrow and spleen, from the same animals used to derive the fibroblasts. This can significantly reduce the number of animals required per study and increase experimental output. In this chapter, we describe the detailed protocols for the isolation, culture, and virus challenge of primary fibroblasts isolated from the ears of adult mice [1, 2].

2 Materials

2.1 Mice

1. Adult mice, 8–10 weeks old (*see* **Notes 1–3**).
2. Surgical tools required: Scissors, forceps, surgical tray.

2.2 Media and Solutions

1. 70 % Ethanol (EtOH).
2. 1× Phosphate-buffered saline (PBS).
3. Kanamycin (10,000 μg).
4. Fetal bovine serum (FBS).
5. Dulbecco's modified Eagle's medium (DMEM).
6. Collagenase (100 mg) and dispase neutral protease from *Bacillus polymyxa* grade II (5 g) (*see* **Note 4**).
7. Streptomycin (10,000 μg) and penicillin (10,000 units) solution.
8. Nonessential amino acids (10 mM).
9. Trypsin–EDTA (0.05 %).
10. Growth media: DMEM, 10 % FBS, 1× nonessential amino acids, 10× penstrep.
11. Serum-free experimental media: DMEM, 1× nonessential amino acids, 1× penstrep.

2.3 Virus Challenge and Interferon β Assays

1. Vesicular stomatitis virus, Orsay (Indiana) (American Type Culture Collection) (*see* **Note 5**).
2. Mouse interferon β ELISA kit.
3. TRIzol reagent.
4. cDNA reverse transcription reagents.
5. Real-time PCR reagents with primer and probe sets to detect mouse *Ifnb1* and *18 s* gene expression.
6. Thermal cycler and real-time quantitative PCR system.

2.4 Tissue Culture Plastics, Materials, and Equipment

1. 12- and 24-well tissue culture-coated plates.
2. 5 ml Serological pipettes.
3. Cell strainers (70 μm).
4. 150 mm tissue-coated Petri dishes.
5. 1.5 ml snap-cap microcentrifuge tubes.
6. 37 °C water bath.
7. 37 °C incubator (5 % CO_2).
8. Refrigerated centrifuge.
9. Inverted microscope (with 10× and 20× objectives).
10. 15 ml conical tubes.
11. Hemacytometer.

3 Methods

3.1 Ear Harvest (See Note 6)

1. Euthanize mice following appropriate institutional guidelines.
2. Remove the left and right pinna from the mouse (*see* **Note** 7) and remove as much excess hair as possible using scissors.
3. Soak each pinna in 70 % EtOH for 5 min and transfer to sterile 1× PBS containing kanamycin (100 μg/ml) (*see* **Note 8**).

3.2 Generation of Primary Cultures

1. Rinse the pinna twice with 1× PBS + kanamycin.
2. Place each pinna in an individual well in a 24-well dish containing 1 ml of growth media.
3. Add the collagenase (4 mg/ml) and protease (4 mg/ml) to enhance cell extraction.
4. Using sterile scissors, mince the pinna in each well as much as possible.
5. Separate the remaining tissue by vigorously pipetting the contents of each well using a 5 ml serological pipette.
6. Incubate the tissue overnight in a 37 °C incubator (*see* **Note 9**).
7. Further dissociate tissue by vigorous pipetting.
8. Pass cells through a cell strainer two times to achieve a single-cell suspension and remove the remaining debris.
9. Pellet the cells by centrifugation at 1,020 × *g* for 5 min.
10. Resuspend the cells in 5 ml of growth media (*see* **Note 10**).
11. Combine the cell suspension for both pinna from individual mice and bring the volume up to 25 ml with growth media. Add the cell suspension to a round 150 mm plate.
12. Grow cells overnight in a 37 °C incubator. This will allow the fibroblasts to adhere. Following the overnight incubation, replace the media with fresh growth media and grow until confluent.

13. Cells should be grown until they become confluent and split densely (*see* **Note 11**).
14. To split cells, remove all supernatant and overlay the cells with 5 ml of 37 °C trypsin–EDTA. Replace the cells in a 37 °C incubator for up to 20 min with light shaking or tapping to induce the cells to release from the plate. Verify that the majority of the cells are no longer attached to the plate by observing under a 10× inverted microscope.
15. Add an equal volume of growth media to the cells and immediately transfer to a 15 ml conical tube. Centrifuge two times at 1,020 × *g* for 5 min, removing the supernatant and resuspending the cells in 10 ml of growth media between each spin.
16. Following the second spin, cells can be quantified using a hemacytometer and replated in 25 ml of growth media.
17. Cells can be split a maximum of three times and maintained for up to 2 weeks (*see* **Note 12**). The cells can be utilized in experiments following the second split.

3.3 Virus Stimulation and Analysis

1. The virus should be prepared and quantified following the supplier's guidelines.
2. Ear fibroblasts can be seeded into individual wells of a 12-well plate at a density of 500,000 cells/well in 1–2 ml of growth media and incubated overnight in a 37 °C incubator (*see* **Note 13**).
3. Following the overnight incubation, the supernatant should be removed and replaced with 1–2 ml of 37 °C serum-free experimental media.
4. The cells should be stimulated with 0.1–1 MOI of VSV (*see* **Note 14**).
5. Ear-derived fibroblasts produce large amounts of secreted proteins, including interferons, chemokines, and cytokines. To evaluate secreted protein levels, supernatants can be harvested over a time course and evaluated using ELISA following the manufacturer's instructions (*see* **Note 15**).
6. To evaluate non-secreted protein production, cells can be lysed directly on the plate using buffers and lysis reagents, such as RIPA buffer, that are appropriate for subsequent western blot analysis.
7. To evaluate gene transcription, 1–2 ml of trypsin–EDTA can be added to each well and incubated at 37 °C for 20 min to induce cell release. Cells can be harvested and collected in a 1.5 ml microcentrifuge tube and centrifuged at 1,020 × *g* for 5 min to pellet the cells. Pelleted cells can then be frozen or lysed for RNA extraction using standard techniques. RNA purification, cDNA amplification, and real-time PCR to evaluate gene expression can be performed using standard techniques.

4 Notes

1. We have exclusively utilized 6–14-week-old C57Bl/6 mice in these assays. It is possible that some aspects of this protocol may need to be adjusted and further optimized when used to derive fibroblasts from mice of different genetic or strain backgrounds.
2. When breeding and identifying mice by ear punch or ear tag, all attempts should be made to limit excessive damage to the ears and preserve the tissue integrity.
3. All studies should be conducted in accordance with the local and institutional animal care and use guidelines and in accord with the prevailing national regulations.
4. Variations of this protocol have successfully utilized collagenase and dispase from other sources. However, some optimization may be required.
5. VSV is infectious and is classified as a BSL-2 pathogen. Materials in this category present a moderate risk to laboratory personnel and should be handled under standard BSL-2 guidelines. Additional pathogen-specific institutional, local, and national regulatory guidelines apply. All infectious materials should be handled under the direct supervision of competent and knowledgeable laboratory personnel. A materials transfer agreement (MTA) with ATCC is required for the use of this pathogen.
6. It is critical that an aseptic environment be maintained at all times during the generation and maintenance of primary cells. Therefore, following ear removal and digestion, all subsequent steps should be carried out under laminar flow conditions. All tools, materials, and surfaces should be sterilized before use and thoroughly cleaned with 70 % ethanol between uses. To prevent cell damage, all solutions should be pre-warmed to 37 °C prior to use. As with other types of primary cells, some level of variability in cell growth and expansion can be expected for each ear fibroblast preparation. These differences may be exaggerated in cells isolated from certain knockout mouse strains. Thus, it is imperative that newly derived fibroblasts be carefully monitored and conditions adjusted as needed to ensure optimal growth [3].
7. In an effort to minimize animal use and optimize time management, it is common to harvest other tissues for primary cell derivation, such as bone marrow and spleen, in addition to the ears.
8. Once in the 1× PBS kanamycin solution, the pinna can be stored overnight at 4 °C or shipped for overnight delivery to collaborators for completion of this protocol.
9. Variations of this protocol have taken advantage of shorter incubation times (minimum recommended length of incubation

is 1 h) in the collagenase and dispase, either with or without serum. However, the protocol presented here results in the maximum digestion of the pinna and typically yields higher cell concentrations when plating.

10. If fungal contamination occurs or is suspected, Fungizone (5 μg/ml) can be added to the resuspended cells prior to plating.
11. Ear fibroblasts should be allowed to grow into dense confluent cultures. The fibroblasts will not grow well if they are split too thin.
12. These protocols are designed for the generation and use of primary ear fibroblasts. While it may be possible to immortalize these cells using protocols similar to those used in the generation of MEFs, we have not attempted this particular manipulation. This is due, in part, to the relative ease of generation for these primary cells.
13. Cell density should be determined empirically depending on the specific growth dynamics of cells generated from genetically modified mice, the inflammatory mediator being assessed, and the kinetics of the specific agent being used to stimulate the cells.
14. VSV is a highly robust model virus that is typically utilized in studies evaluating the production of type I interferon. However, many viruses are cell type specific and/or require specific modifications to the local environment prior to use. For example, some viruses require low levels of trypsin to be present in order to facilitate infection. Therefore, the specific conditions associated with the virus challenge should be determined empirically. It should also be noted that live virus will be present in sample preparations. Thus, additional steps may be required to inactivate the virus, including heat or UV inactivation.
15. We routinely observe high levels of specific cytokines, such as IL-6, under naïve conditions. This contributes to high background levels and may impact subsequent studies focused on these specific cytokines.

References

1. Shao C, Deng L, Henegariu O, Liang L, Raikwar N, Sahota A, Stambrook PJ, Tischfield JA (1999) Mitotic recombination produces the majority of recessive fibroblast variants in heterozygous mice. Proc Natl Acad Sci U S A 96:9230–9235
2. Allen IC, Moore CB, Schneider M, Lei Y, Davis BK, Scull MA, Gris D, Roney KE, Zimmermann AG, Bowzard JB, Ranjan P, Monroe KM, Pickles RJ, Sambhara S, Ting JP (2011) NLRX1 protein attenuates inflammatory responses to infection by interfering with the RIG-I-MAVS and TRAF6-NF-kappaB signaling pathways. Immunity 34:854–865
3. Garfield AS (2010) Derivation of primary mouse embryonic fibroblast (PMEF) cultures. Methods Mol Biol 633:19–27

Chapter 9

Bone Marrow-Derived Dendritic Cells

Kelly Roney

Abstract

While much is understood about dendritic cells and their role in the immune system, the study of these cells is critical to gain a more complete understanding of their function. Dendritic cell isolation from mouse body tissues can be difficult and the number of cells isolated small. This protocol describes the growth of large number of dendritic cells from the culture of mouse bone marrow cells. The dendritic cells grown in culture facilitate experiments that may require large number of dendritic cells without great expense or use of large number of mice.

Key words Dendritic cell, Mouse, Bone marrow, GM-CSF, IL-4

1 Introduction

Dendritic cells are found in many areas of the body, including skin, spleen, lung, and blood. Studies of dendritic cells are critical for understanding many immune processes, such as antigen uptake and T cell activation [1–3]. The study of ex vivo dendritic cells can be difficult due to the small number of cells that can be isolated. Thus, the ability to grow large number of dendritic cells derived from mouse bone marrow has facilitated many studies that would have otherwise been difficult [4]. The protocol described in this chapter outlines a method of generating large number of dendritic cells from mouse bone marrow [5–7].

2 Materials

1. Phosphate-buffered saline (PBS).
2. 70 % Ethanol.
3. Roswell Park Memorial Institute media (RPMI)-1640.

Irving C. Allen (ed.), *Mouse Models of Innate Immunity: Methods and Protocols*, Methods in Molecular Biology, vol. 1031, DOI 10.1007/978-1-62703-481-4_9, © Springer Science+Business Media, LLC 2013

4. Complete RPMI: 500 ml of RPMI-1640, 5.5×10^5 mol/l of 2-mercaptoethanol, 25 mM/l of HEPES, 100 U/ml of penicillin, 100 μg/ml of streptomycin sulfate, 50 ml of heat-inactivated fetal bovine serum (use serum of sufficient grade for primary cell culture).
5. Buffered ammonium chloride (ACK) lysis buffer: Add 4.14 g of NH_4Cl, 0.5 g of $KHCO_3$, 18.8 mg of Na_2 EDTA into 300 ml of double-distilled water (or an equivalent) and stir to dissolve. Bring the solution up to 500 ml using double-distilled water (or an equivalent) and adjust the pH to 7.2–7.4 with 1 N HCl. Filter the solution with a 70 μm nylon filter and store at room temperature.
6. Mouse granulocyte-macrophage colony-stimulating factor (GM-CSF).
7. Mouse interleukin-4 (IL-4).
8. Mouse tumor necrosis factor (TNF alpha).
9. 100 mm × 20 mm culture plate without tissue-culture treatment.
10. 6-well culture plate without tissue-culture treatment.
11. Sterilized 4 in. (or similar size) forceps.
12. Sterilized 4 in. (or similar size) scissors.
13. Sterile paper towels or other absorbent materials.
14. Sterile needles: 22 gauge × 1 in. (*see* **Note 1**).
15. 1 ml sterile syringe (*see* **Note 1**).
16. 50 ml conical sterile polypropylene tubes.
17. 15 ml conical polypropylene tubes.

3 Methods

3.1 Bone Marrow Isolation (See Note 2)

1. Euthanize the mouse according to local animal care and use committee guidelines and regulations. Bone marrow should be harvested immediately following euthanization for best yield.
2. Remove the skin from the abdomen down. Remove the hind legs by blunt dissection. Separate the femur from the tibia by cutting the connection point with scissors (*see* **Note 3**).
3. Remove the muscle and as much connective tissue as possible from the femurs and tibias by firmly grasping the top of the bone with two sets of forceps held in an upside down "V" while resting the bottom of the bone on sterilized paper towels. Slide the forceps down the bone while firmly grasping the bone, removing the muscle and tissue. Muscle and tissue remaining at the bottom of the bone may be removed with scissors.

4. Place the harvested bone into a 100 mm non-tissue culture-treated plate on ice filled with PBS until all bones are harvested (*see* **Note 4**).
5. While grasping the bone with forceps, remove the epiphyses by cutting the tips of the bone with scissors (*see* **Note 5**).
6. Fill a 100 mm non-tissue culture-treated plate with cold complete RPMI (enough to cover the bottom). Prepare a 1 ml syringe by fitting with a 27 gauge needle and filing with cold complete RPMI.
7. Using the prefilled syringe, remove the bone marrow from the bone by placing the tip of the needle in the bone while grasping the bone with forceps and injecting complete RPMI to flush out the marrow into the petri dish containing complete RPMI (*see* **Note 6**).
8. Completely remove the bone marrow from all four leg bones and combine into a single petri dish. Using the same syringe used to flush the bones, gently disperse any clumps of bone marrow by pulling the media and bone marrow into the syringe and releasing.
9. Place a 70 μm cell strainer atop a 50 ml conical tube. Pipette the RPMI/bone marrow cell solution from the petri dish through the cell strainer.
10. Remove the plunger from the syringe, and use the rubber tip of the plunger to disperse any bone marrow or tissue clumps left in the strainer. Rinse the cell strainer with complete RPMI (*see* **Note** 7).
11. Spin the media/cell mixture at 13,523 × *g* at 4 °C for 5 min to pellet the cells.
12. Discard the media by gently tilting the tube and pouring off the media into a waste disposal beaker. Recap the tube and gently tap to break up the cell pellet. Place the tube on ice.
13. Add 1.0 ml of cell lysis solution to the cells and gently tap the tube with your finger to mix the lysis solution for 30–60 s.
14. Immediately add 50 ml of ice-cold PBS to dilute the lysis buffer.
15. Centrifuge the PBS/cell mixture at 13,523 × *g* at 4 °C for 5 min to pellet the cells. Remove the PBS by gently tilting the tube and pouring off the PBS into a waste disposal beaker. Recap and gently tap the tube with your finger to break up the cell pellet.
16. Resuspend the cell pellet in 50 ml of ice-cold PBS to wash the cells. Centrifuge the PBS/cell mixture at 13,523 × *g* at 4 °C for 5 min to pellet the cells.

17. Resuspend the cells in 10 ml of cold complete RPMI, and place on ice. Remove 100 μl of the cell suspension and count the cells. Bone marrow harvested from two tibias and two fibias should yield approximately 70×10^6 cells. Health, age, and transplant status of the mouse may affect bone marrow yields [8].

3.2 Dendritic Cell Culture

1. Day 0: Plate 2×10^6 cells in 20 ml of media with 20 ng/ml of GM-CSF onto a 100 mm non-tissue culture-treated culture plate (*see* **Notes 8** and **9**).
2. Day 3: Add 20 ml of media with GM-CSF to bring the final concentration of GM-CSF for the whole culture (a total of 40 ml) to 10 ng/ml.
3. Day 6: Remove 20 ml from the plate. Centrifuge to recover the cells, discard the supernatant, and resuspend the pellet in 20 ml of complete RPMI. Add GM-CSF and IL-4 so that the final concentration of the entire culture is 10 ng/ml of GM-CSF and 10 ng/ml of IL-4 (*see* **Note 10**).
4. Day 8: Repeat **step 3**; only use 5 ng/ml of GM-CSF and 10 ng/ml of IL-4 for the total culture concentration.
5. Day 10: Harvest the dendritic cells, which will be floating or lightly adherent in the culture. To harvest, remove the media containing the DCs and transfer to a 50 ml conical tube. Plates can be rinsed gently with warmed PBS to remove the lightly adherent cells. Avoid harvesting the adherent cells.
6. Dendritic cells may be used on day 10 or may be further matured (*see* **Note 11**).

3.3 Maturation

1. Day 10: Wash the cells twice in cold PBS and count. Resuspend cells in complete RPMI media at a concentration of 1×10^6 cells/ml. Add 1 ml of cells to each well of a 6-well bacterial culture plate (*see* **Notes 11** and **12**).
2. Add 1 ml of complete RPMI to each well so that the concentration of the culture is 5 ng/ml of GM-CSF, 5 ng/ml of IL-4, and 20 ng/ml of TNF (*see* **Note 11**).
3. Day 10 + 1: The following day add 1.0 ml of media with TNF to each well so that the concentration in the entire culture is 10 ng/ml. Harvest the cells for use the following day (*see* **Note 11**).
4. Day 10 + 2: The mature dendritic cells will be loosely adherent. To harvest, remove the media from the culture and transfer to a 15 ml conical tube. Add cold PBS to the culture plate and gently loosen cells from the plate with a cell scraper. Add the cold PBS–cell mixture to the media in the 15 ml conical tube, pellet the cells by centrifugation, and wash in cold PBS to remove residual cytokines (*see* **Note 11**).

4 Notes

1. Needle length and gauge size may be varied to meet individual preferences and/or hand size. A 5 or a 10 ml syringe may also be used instead of the 1 ml syringe to meet individual preferences.
2. All procedures should be carried out at room temperature unless otherwise specified. All procedures except centrifugation should be performed in a laminar flow hood or other types of hood sufficient for tissue culture. Tissue culture techniques should be utilized throughout the procedure.
3. A beaker filled with 70 % ethanol can be used to dip forceps and scissors. This technique is a good way to remove hair or tissue from the tools during bone marrow isolation.
4. Bones may be sterilized by submerging in cold 70 % ethanol for 2 min in a 100 mm bacterial culture plate and then rinsing two times by submerging bones in a dish with cold PBS for 2 min to rinse away the ethanol. We have not found this step necessary if good tissue culture techniques are used for bone marrow isolation.
5. If bone marrow material is a limiting factor, the epiphyses can be cut into pieces in compete media in a petri dish. The resulting bone marrow cells can be isolated by running the complete media and bone through a 70 μm size cell strainer.
6. The bone should turn a brighter white and more translucent as the marrow is flushed. Removal of the syringe to the opposite end of the bone, or an additional flush of complete media, is often necessary. If necessary, the syringe can be refilled from the media in the marrow collection petri dish.
7. Cells may be placed on ice at this stage for 1–2 h if complete media is used.
8. Count bone marrow cells carefully. Overplating may result in over-proliferated cells that will not differentiate into dendritic cells.
9. If a smaller number of cells are desired from a single plate, cells may be grown in 100 × 20 mm non-tissue culture-treated plates in 10 ml of media. Adjust all steps forward to a starting amount of 10 ml of media.
10. For the best results, warm the resuspended cells to 37 °C before returning to the culture plate to prevent cooling of the cell culture plate.
11. Dendritic cells that are in a more immature state may be better for some experiments, such as antigen uptake assays, whereas other experiments may require a more mature cell that has received more cytokine stimulation.

12. Alternative day 10 for larger cell cultures: Suspend cells at 1×10^6 cells per ml and plate 5 ml on a 100 mm non-tissue culture-treated plate. Then add 5 ml of media. The final cytokine concentrations should be 5 ng/ml of GM-CSF, 5 ng/ml of IL-4, and 20 ng/ml of TNF. Alternative day 10 + 1: Add 10 ml of media with 10 ng/ml of TNF for the entire culture. Harvest cells on alternative D10 + 2.

References

1. Altfeld M, Fadda L, Frleta D, Bhardwaj N (2011) DCs and NK cells: critical effectors in the immune response to HIV-1. Nat Rev Immunol 11:176–186
2. Bousso P (2008) T-cell activation by dendritic cells in the lymph node: lessons from the movies. Nat Rev Immunol 8:675–684
3. Roy RM, Klein BS (2012) Dendritic cells in antifungal immunity and vaccine design. Cell Host Microbe 11:436–446
4. Inaba K, Inaba M, Romani N, Aya H, Deguchi M, Ikehara S, Muramatsu S, Steinman RM (1992) Generation of large number of dendritic cells from mouse bone marrow cultures supplemented with granulocyte/macrophage colony-stimulating factor. J Exp Med 176:1693–1702
5. Lutz MB, Kukutsch N, Ogilvie AL, Rossner S, Koch F, Romani N, Schuler G (1999) An advanced culture method for generating large quantities of highly pure dendritic cells from mouse bone marrow. J Immunol Methods 223:77–92
6. Van Deventer HW, Serody JS, Mckinnon KP, Clements C, Brickey WJ, Ting JP (2002) Transfection of macrophage inflammatory protein 1 alpha into B16 F10 melanoma cells inhibits growth of pulmonary metastases but not subcutaneous tumors. J Immunol 169:1634–1639
7. Wong AW, Brickey WJ, Taxman DJ, Van Deventer HW, Reed W, Gao JX, Zheng P, Liu Y, Li P, Blum JS, Mckinnon KP, Ting JP (2003) CIITA-regulated plexin-A1 affects T-cell-dendritic cell interactions. Nat Immunol 4:891–898
8. Lutz MB, Rossner S (2007) Factors influencing the generation of murine dendritic cells from bone marrow: the special role of fetal calf serum. Immunobiology 212:855–862

Chapter 10

Measuring T Cell Function in Innate Immune Models

Brianne R. Barker

Abstract

Innate immune responses often result in the activation and modulation of T lymphocyte function. Analysis of T lymphocytes in mouse models of innate immunity can allow understanding of the links between the innate and adaptive immune systems. Other T lymphocyte populations display innate-like functions. Isolation of T cells and evaluation of their surface proteins can provide data on T cell activation, as can an analysis of T cell proliferation. Further insight may be obtained by examining cytokine production via intracellular cytokine staining or ELISPOT to determine T cell function. This chapter describes methods for T cell isolation, measurement of surface protein expression, T cell proliferation, intracellular cytokine staining, and ELISPOT.

Key words Flow cytometry, Intracellular cytokine staining, ELISPOT, CFSE

1 Introduction

Although T lymphocytes are considered adaptive immune cells, measurement of ex vivo T cell responses can play an important role in elucidating the innate immune response. Innate immune cells and molecules play an integral role in the activation and differentiation of adaptive immune cells [1–6]. Thus, investigators are often interested in T cell function as a way to fully demonstrate the link between innate and adaptive immunity. In addition, innate-like lymphocytes such as NKT cells and γδ T cells can be functionally characterized using the methods developed for classical T cells [7–10]. In either case, methods to characterize T cell number and function ex vivo are key to describing the potency of an innate immune response.

To perform any of the T cell analyses that follow, one must first isolate these cells from the experimental animal. Standard protocols for the isolation of leukocytes from murine peripheral blood or secondary lymphoid organs are included below. Examination of T cell populations from these organs allows for the assessment of

Irving C. Allen (ed.), *Mouse Models of Innate Immunity: Methods and Protocols*, Methods in Molecular Biology, vol. 1031, DOI 10.1007/978-1-62703-481-4_10,

immune responses occurring systemically or in draining lymph nodes. As T cell effector function often takes place away from these sites, it may be of interest to isolate T cells from other anatomic locations as well. In addition, some of the innate-like lymphocyte populations may be commonly found in locations including the liver, gastrointestinal tract, and skin, making these tissues of potential interest. Specific details for the isolation of T cells from other sites are unique and are not presented here. It should be noted that many of these protocols may involve collagenase digestion or other lengthy incubation periods that may adversely affect the surface proteins expressed by cells. These manipulations may alter the cells' functions and they should be optimized with care. Cells isolated using the secondary lymphoid organ protocols described below or other tissues may be used in the assays to evaluate T cell function presented later in the chapter although the number of cells isolated from each tissue may vary considerably. Secondary lymphoid organs, particularly spleen, result in the isolation of a large number of cells that allows one to perform multiple assays described with one experimental animal. All of the protocols provided result in the isolation of total leukocytes, as do most of the available protocols for cell isolation from other tissues, and this fact should be remembered when performing subsequent assays. The use of T cell-specific stimuli or flow cytometric analysis of T cell-specific surface proteins is often necessary to ensure specificity of the responses measured. Magnetic bead-based selection protocols may be used to isolate T cells from these bulk cell populations, but these protocols should be based on negative selection to avoid background activation of T cells before analysis. These selection procedures should be tested to ensure that they result in high yields of unactivated T cells.

The simplest way to evaluate T cells is via surface staining and flow cytometric analysis. This technique allows for the simple measurement of the proportion of T cells or specific T cell subsets among the isolated leukocytes, possibly from an effector site, or measurement of absolute cell numbers when combined with cell counts. The expression of specific trafficking molecules or activation molecules is often of interest as well and can provide insight into T cells' functional capabilities or differentiation state. This simple method also underlies some of the more complex protocols that follow. T cell activation can also be measured by examining T cell proliferation, here presented as the measurement of carboxyfluorescein diacetate succinimidyl ester (CFSE) dilution using a flow cytometer. In this technique, isolated cells are labeled with the cell-permeant dye CFSE, which labels all cellular proteins. These cells are then stimulated with peptide antigen or other T cell-specific stimuli in in vitro culture. At varying time points following stimulation, cells are removed from culture and analyzed by flow cytometry and CFSE fluorescence is measured. Lower levels of fluorescence indicate more rounds of cell division. This method has an advantage over other proliferation assays, including ^{3}H-thymidine incorporation or MTT metabolism assays in that surface staining for other T cell-specific markers can be used to ensure that the proliferation of T cells is being measured or to allow measurement of proliferation and surface markers of T cell function simultaneously.

Many T cell subpopulations, particularly helper T cell populations, are commonly distinguished based on cytokine production. Two methods to measure cytokine production are presented here: intracellular cytokine staining (using flow cytometry) and ELISPOT. These methods allow for measurement of cytokines from specific cell populations or following specific stimulation, unlike cytokine ELISAs of serum, which provide information about systemic cytokine levels. Cytokine ELISAs are available from many manufacturers and can often be performed according to their specifications. Both intracellular cytokine staining and ELISPOT can be performed on cells taken directly ex vivo or on cells that are stimulated with a specific antigen to measure in vitro cytokine production. Intracellular cytokine staining involves the utilization of cell permeabilization techniques and flow cytometry. This technique can be combined with cell surface staining to allow for the determination of cytokine production from specific T cell subsets or for the conservation of experimental animals. Permeabilization techniques can also be modified for the detection of signal transduction molecules [11]. Intracellular staining has the advantage of providing data regarding the specific cell subpopulations responsible for cytokine production as well as the relative amount of cytokine production, which is based on brightness. ELISPOT involves culturing cells in multiscreen plates and evaluating the secreted cytokines. Secreted cytokines can be measured via an ELISA-like protocol. ELISPOT has the advantage of providing data pertaining to the number of cells in a population that are producing a cytokine of interest. Based on their sensitivities, each of these two techniques may be more suited to measuring the levels of different cytokines.

2 Materials

2.1 Harvesting Leukocytes from Peripheral Blood

1. Mice to be assessed.
2. Blood collection media: RPMI 1640 with 40 U/ml of heparan sulfate (*see* **Notes 1** and **2**).
3. Lympholyte M or other types of Ficoll (*see* **Note 3**).
4. ACK buffer (*see* **Note 3**): Add nine parts 0.16 M NH_4Cl to one part of 0.17 M Tris base pH 7.65, then adjust the pH of the resulting solution to 7.2, and sterile filter.
5. 15 ml polystyrene conical tubes.

6. Equipment for the collection of mouse blood (*see* **Note 4**).
7. Refrigerated centrifuge capable of spinning 15 ml conical tubes.
8. Sterile and pyrogen-free PBS with 2 % fetal bovine serum (sterile filtered) (*see* **Notes 1** and **5**).

2.2 Harvesting Leukocytes from Spleen and Lymph Nodes

1. Mice to be assessed.
2. Equipment to euthanize mice (*see* **Note 6**).
3. Sterile surgical instruments: Forceps, scissors, Jeweler's forceps that may be particularly useful to isolate lymph nodes, dissection tray, and dissection pins.
4. 70 % ethanol.
5. Spleen/lymph node collection media: Hank's Balanced Salt Solution with 4 % fetal bovine serum and 10 mM HEPES (sterile filtered; *see* **Note 1**).
6. Lympholyte M or other types of Ficoll (*see* **Note 3**).
7. ACK buffer (*see* **Note 3**): Add nine parts 0.16 M NH_4Cl to one part of 0.17 M Tris base pH 7.65, then adjust the pH of the resulting solution to 7.2, and sterile filter.
8. 15 ml polystyrene conical tubes.
9. Refrigerated centrifuge capable of spinning 15 ml conical tubes.
10. Sterile and pyrogen-free PBS with 2 % fetal bovine serum (sterile filtered) (*see* **Note 5**).
11. Hemocytometer and trypan blue (optional).
12. Light microscope.
13. 100 μm cell strainer per mouse (*see* **Note 7**).
14. Plunger from a 1cc syringe per mouse (*see* **Note 7**).
15. Petri dishes or 6-well tissue culture plates (*see* **Note 7**).
16. R10 media: RPMI 1640 plus 10 % fetal bovine serum, 1 % MEM nonessential amino acids, 0.1 % β-mercaptoethanol, 1 % sodium pyruvate, and 1 % penicillin/streptomycin.

2.3 Surface Staining

1. 12 × 75 mm 5 ml test tubes (*see* **Note 8**).
2. Centrifuge capable of spinning 5 ml conical tubes.
3. Sterile and pyrogen-free PBS with 2 % fetal bovine serum (sterile filtered) (*see* **Notes 1** and **5**).
4. Ca- and Mg-free PBS or Ca- and Mg-free PBS with 2 % formaldehyde (*see* **Note 9**).
5. Flow cytometer and flow cytometry analysis software.
6. Fluorescence-conjugated antibodies against surface molecules of interest.
7. Vortex.

2.4 Proliferation

1. All materials listed above for surface staining.
2. Hank's Balanced Salt Solution.
3. 15 ml conical tubes.
4. CFSE: Generate a stock solution of 1 mM CFSE in DMSO. This solution is frozen at −20 °C (*see* **Note 10**).
5. R10 media: RPMI 1640 plus 10 % fetal bovine serum, 1 % MEM nonessential amino acids, 0.1 % β-mercaptoethanol, 1 % sodium pyruvate, and 1 % penicillin/streptomycin.
6. Rat IL-2.
7. 37 °C incubator.
8. Specific antigenic peptide or overlapping peptide pools.
9. Anti-CD3ε (low endotoxin, azide free).
10. Round-bottom 96-well tissue culture plates.

2.5 Intracellular Cytokine Staining

1. All materials listed above for surface staining.
2. Stimulation media (*see* **Note 11**): RPMI 1640 plus 10 % fetal bovine serum, 1 % MEM nonessential amino acids, 0.1 % β-mercaptoethanol, 1 % sodium pyruvate, and 1 % penicillin/streptomycin plus 2 μg/ml anti-CD28 (azide free) and 2 μg/ml anti-CD49d (azide free).
3. Fluorescence-conjugated antibodies against cytokines or other intracellular molecules of interest (*see* **Note 12**).
4. Phorbol 12-myristate 13-acetate (PMA).
5. Ionomycin.
6. Specific antigenic peptide or overlapping peptide pools.
7. Cytofix/Cytoperm solution (BD Biosciences) (*see* **Note 12**).
8. Brefeldin A or Monensin (BD Biosciences).
9. 37 °C incubator.
10. Perm/Wash Buffer (BD Biosciences) (*see* **Note 12**).

2.6 ELISPOT

1. PMA.
2. Ionomycin.
3. Specific antigenic peptide or overlapping peptide pools.
4. 96 well multiscreen plates (Millipore Immobilon-P PVDF plates).
5. Ca- and Mg-free PBS (sterile and pyrogen free).
6. Anti-cytokine antibodies for coating plates (i.e., anti-IFN-γ).
7. PBS containing 0.25 % Tween 20 (PBS/Tween).
8. PBS containing 10 % fetal bovine serum.
9. Multichannel pipette.
10. 96-well plate washer (optional).

11. 37 °C incubator.
12. Distilled water.
13. Biotinylated anti-cytokine antibody (i.e., biotinylated anti-IFN-γ).
14. Streptavidin alkaline phosphatase.
15. Nitroblue tetrazolium (NBT)/5-bromo-4-chloro-3-indolylphosphate (BCIP) chromogen solution (Pierce).
16. Automated ELISPOT reader and image-processing software. Commonly used readers are from Hitech Instruments or the CTL Analyzer (CTL Analyzers LLC, Cleveland, OH). Common image-processing software include Image-Pro Plus (Media Cybernetics, Des Moines, Iowa) or CTL software (CTL Analyzers LLC, Cleveland, OH).

3 Methods

3.1 Harvesting Leukocytes from Peripheral Blood

1. Fill one 15 ml conical tube with 3 ml of blood collection media per mouse (*see* **Notes 2** and **4**).
2. Collect peripheral blood and immediately place in a 15 ml tube with blood collection media.
3. Underlay 1 ml of Lympholyte M with a 2 ml pipette (*see* **Notes 3** and **13**).
4. Centrifuge at 1,875 × *g* for 20 min at 10 °C without brake.
5. Remove the cell layer from the Lympholyte M and add to 10 ml of PBS/2 % FCS in a new 15 ml conical tube.
6. Centrifuge at 500 × *g* for 10 min.
7. Aspirate and resuspend the resulting cell pellet for downstream applications (*see* **Note 14**).

3.2 Harvesting Leukocytes from Spleen and Lymph Nodes

1. Fill one 15 ml conical tube with 5 ml of spleen/lymph node collection media per mouse, per organ to be isolated.
2. Euthanize mice one at a time and isolate the spleen or the lymph nodes from each mouse immediately after sacrifice (*see* **Note 6**). Immediately place the organ in a 15 ml tube with spleen/lymph node collection media. Collect all organs from all mice and place them on ice before proceeding to the next step.
3. Gently homogenize the spleen or the lymph node through the 100 μm cell strainer into a small Petri dish using the plunger from the 1cc syringe until a single-cell suspension is produced. Pipette the single-cell suspension into a 15 ml conical tube. Wash the strainer, plunger, and dish with 5 ml of mouse R10 and add to the same conical tube (*see* **Note 7**).
4. Centrifuge at 500 × *g* for 5 min.

5. Underlay 1 ml of Lympholyte M with a 2 ml pipette (*see* **Notes 3** and **13**).
6. Centrifuge at 1,875 × *g* for 20 min at 10 °C without the brake.
7. Remove the cell layer from the Lympholyte M and add to 10 ml of PBS/2 % FCS in a new 15 ml conical tube.
8. Centrifuge at 500 × *g* for 10 min.
9. Aspirate and resuspend the resulting cell pellet in 10 ml of 2 % PBS/FCS and count the cells for downstream applications (*see* **Note 14**).

3.3 Surface Staining

1. Transfer at least 1×10^6 cells per sample to 12 × 75 mm 5 ml test tubes. Adjust the volume to 100 μl with PBS/2 % FCS. Also, transfer at least 1×10^6 cells to a 12 × 75 mm 5 ml test tube to use for unstained controls, single-color controls, and possibly FMO controls. Adjust the volume to 100 μl with PBS/2 % FCS (*see* **Note 15**).
2. Prepare a cocktail containing the appropriate amounts of each cell surface-staining antibody before staining and add this cocktail to the cells to stain (*see* **Notes 16** and **17**). Add individual diluted antibodies to single-color control tubes. Vortex all samples and incubate them for 30 min on ice in the dark.
3. Add 3 ml of PBS/2 % FCS to each tube and centrifuge at 500 × *g* for 5 min to wash.
4. Aspirate and resuspend the cells in 500 μl of PBS or PBS/2 % formaldehyde while vortexing to reduce clumping (*see* **Note 9**). Store the cells at 4 °C and analyze the cells using the flow cytometer.

3.4 Proliferation

1. Add 10×10^6 cells to a 15 ml conical tube. Wash the cells twice with 10 ml of HBSS (*see* **Notes 18** and **19**). Resuspend 10×10^6 cells in 900 μl of HBSS with no serum. Be sure to set up additional cells for unstained and single-color controls for later flow cytometry analysis.
2. Incubate the cells in HBSS with 1 μM of CFSE for 30 min at 37 °C. Mix by shaking the tube vigorously, but not vortexing.
3. After the 30-min incubation, wash the cells twice with R10 media (*see* **Note 18**).
4. Resuspend the cells at 1.5×10^6 cells/ml in R10 media. Plate the cells in a round-bottom 96-well plate at 200 μl/well. Add 100 ng/ml of peptide antigen or anti-CD3 as a control (*see* **Note 20**). Be sure to set up additional wells without the peptide as a control.
5. Add 25 U/ml of rat IL-2 on day 2 of the culture (*see* **Note 21**).
6. Take cells for staining as desired (anytime between day 0 and day 8) and apply the surface staining protocol as above.

3.5 Intracellular Cytokine Staining

1. Transfer at least 4×10^6 cells per sample to 12×75 mm 5 ml test tubes (*see* **Note 8**). Adjust the volume to 500 μl of stimulation media. Also transfer at least 4×10^6 cells to a 12×75 mm 5 ml test tube for controls for staining per experiment (unstained control, single-color controls) and controls for stimulation per sample (unstimulated, antigen stimulated, and PMA/ionomycin stimulated). Adjust the volume to 500 μl with stimulation media (*see* **Notes 11**, **15**, and **20**).
2. Add 1 μl of Golgi-stop to each sample. Add 1 μg of antigenic peptide or peptide pool to each sample to be stimulated with antigen. Add 0.5 μg of PMA and 2.5 μg of ionomycin to each positive control (PMA/ionomycin sample).
3. Vortex the cells, place the caps on loosely on the tubes, and incubate the samples for 6 h at 37 °C (*see* **Note 22**).
4. Add 3 ml of PBS/2 % FCS to each tube and centrifuge at $500 \times g$ for 5 min to wash. Adjust the volume to 100 μl of PBS/2 % FCS.
5. Prepare a cocktail containing the appropriate amounts of each of the surface-staining antibodies before staining and add this cocktail to the cells to stain (*see* **Note 17**). Add individual diluted antibodies to single-color control tubes. Vortex all samples and incubate them for 30 min on ice in the dark.
6. Add 3 ml of PBS/2 % FCS to each tube and centrifuge at $500 \times g$ for 5 min to wash (*see* **Note 17**).
7. Vortex each sample. While vortexing, add 500 μl of Cytofix/Cytoperm. Incubate at room temperature for 45 min (*see* **Note 22**).
8. Add 2 ml of perm/wash buffer and centrifuge at $800 \times g$ for 7 min to wash. Aspirate the supernatant and wash with another 2 ml of perm/wash buffer.
9. Vortex each sample. Prepare a cocktail containing the appropriate amounts of all of the intracellular staining antibodies before staining and add this cocktail to the cells to stain (*see* **Notes 12** and **17**). Vortex all samples and incubate them for 30 min on ice in the dark.
10. Add 2 ml of perm/wash buffer. Centrifuge the samples at $800 \times g$ for 7 min to wash.
11. Aspirate the supernatant and resuspend the cells in 500 μl of PBS or PBS/2 % formaldehyde while vortexing to reduce clumping (*see* **Note 9**). Store the cells at 4 °C until ready for analysis on the flow cytometer.

3.6 ELISPOT

1. Coat 96-well multiscreen plates with 100 μl per well of 5 μg/ml of anti-cytokine antibody diluted in PBS. Incubate the plates overnight.

2. Wash plates three times with PBS containing 0.25 % Tween 20 (PBS/Tween) (*see* **Note 23**).
3. Add 200 μl per well of PBS containing 10 % fetal bovine serum to block the plates. Incubate the plates for 2 h at room temperature.
4. Add 2×10^5 cells and the appropriate antigenic peptides (1 μg/ml) or other stimuli to each well. It is advisable to set up triplicate wells for each condition. Unstimulated cells should also be included in the assay to allow for an assessment of background cytokine production. Incubate the plates for 18 h at 37 °C (*see* **Note 20**).
5. Wash the plates nine times with PBS/Tween and once with distilled water.
6. Add 2 μg of biotinylated anti-cytokine antibody diluted in PBS and bring the volume of each well up to a total volume of 100 μl. Incubate for 2 h at room temperature.
7. Wash the plate six times with PBS/Tween.
8. Incubate the plates with a 1:500 dilution (100 μl total volume per well, dilute in PBS) of streptavidin-alkaline phosphatase for 2.5 h.
9. Wash the plate five times with PBS/Tween and once with PBS only.
10. Develop the plates by adding NBT/BCIP chromogen solution. Stop the reaction once color has developed with tap water and air-dry plates.
11. Read the plates with an automated ELISPOT reader and quantitate the number of spots apparent using appropriate software. Data from an ELISPOT assay are usually expressed as spot-forming cells (SFC) per 10^6 cells added to the well and compared to background levels seen in unstimulated cells.

4 Notes

1. Prepare all solutions using ultrapure water and pyrogen-free, tissue culture-grade reagents. Store all reagents at 4 °C unless indicated otherwise. Pay careful attention to waste disposal recommendations of your institution; some prepackaged kits or reagents contain preservatives that may require special collection and disposal. We perform all assays using sterile technique in a laminar flow hood, although terminal assays in which cells will not be cultured may be performed on a bench top. Be sure to wear appropriate personal protective equipment throughout the procedure.

2. Blood should be collected in the presence of anticoagulant; however, we have used anticoagulants other than heparin in our blood collection media with generally good results. Calcium chelators, such as EDTA, can adversely affect some functional assays including intracellular cytokine staining and should be tested carefully.
3. We use Lympholyte M as a standard way of separating peripheral blood mononuclear cells from other cell types found in peripheral blood or secondary lymphoid organs. We find that this technique provides the cleanest cell population without debris that can cause problems in cytometry. Instead of using Lympholyte M or another type of ficoll, it is possible to lyse the red blood cells in a single-cell suspension with NH_4Cl lysis buffer (ACK). Further, some tissues, particularly spleen, contain large number of red blood cells and cell preparations from these tissues may be improved by adding an ACK lysis step following Lympholyte treatment. The following is an alternative ACK lysis protocol: (a) Centrifuge heparinized blood or single-cell suspension generated from spleen or lymph node. (b) Approximately 5 ml of ACK solution should be added to the cell pellet. The specific amount will vary based on the number of cells. (c) Invert tubes to mix well and incubate for approximately 3 min. The amount of time will also vary based on the number of cells and tissue. Do not overlyse. (d) Centrifuge tubes immediately to remove ACK buffer. Overlysis of cells can cause problems with surface staining, functional assays, or can result in poor cell yield.
4. Appropriate techniques for the collection of mouse blood vary among institutions and IACUC committees. We have successfully used blood obtained via retroorbital (generally disfavored among IACUC committees), submandibular, and cardiac puncture routes. Submandibular blood collection utilizing Goldenrod Animal Lancets can be performed on live mice and allows the investigator to follow the same mice throughout the course of disease. However, submandibular blood collection results in smaller volumes of blood for experimentation. Blood volume may be replaced with Ringer's lactate solution. Blood collection via cardiac puncture results in larger volumes of blood for experimentation, but is a terminal procedure and does not allow the mice to be followed at multiple time points.
5. Throughout this protocol, PBS with 2 % fetal bovine serum can be substituted with PBS with BSA.
6. Appropriate techniques for mouse euthanasia vary among institutions and IACUC committees.
7. There are multiple methods of dissociating spleens and lymph nodes to generate single-cell suspensions. We tend to use

syringe plungers and disposable cell strainers in either Petri dishes or wells of 6-well tissue culture plates. We have also used syringe plungers or autoclavable glass rods with autoclavable mesh screens in a similar fashion to the method described here for homogenizing spleens between two frosted glass slides.

8. Flow cytometry staining and analysis are traditionally performed in 5 ml test tubes. However, the use of these tubes may be cumbersome when staining large number of samples. Alternatively, we have stained cells in round-bottom 96-well plates or strips of PCR tubes. Either of these methods allows for the use of a multichannel pipette. Both alternatives require additional wash steps, as cells cannot be washed with large volumes of liquid. A centrifuge capable of spinning 96-well plates is also necessary. Cells can then be transferred into 5 ml test tubes for analysis or may be analyzed directly in a 96-well plate if appropriate flow cytometer hardware is available.

9. We fix our samples for flow cytometry with formaldehyde as a standard procedure. However, cell fixation is not necessary provided that there are no biosafety concerns and the samples will be analyzed on a flow cytometer immediately. In this case, cells can be resuspended in PBS alone. Formaldehyde fixation can alter some fluorophores, so fixed and unfixed samples should not be compared.

10. When attached to proteins, the emission and excitation peaks of CFSE are 492 and 517 nm and it is typically read in the FITC channel. CFSE should be carefully titrated to ensure that spillover into other channels does not occur. Similar compounds with different emission and excitation peaks (i.e., CellTrace™ Violet Cell Proliferation Kit (Molecular Probes)) have been developed and allow good results.

11. Stimulation media is the R10 media listed above with the addition of purified, azide-free anti-CD28 and anti-CD49d antibodies. These antibodies allow for co-stimulation of T cells during antigenic stimulation and result in optimal cytokine production. The specific antibodies used in this stimulation media, particularly with regard to the use of CD49d, vary among investigators. If direct ex vivo cytokine analysis is desired, this media is not necessary.

12. The protocol presented here is specific for staining for intracellular cytokines and uses the detergent for saponin for cell permeabilization. The BD CytoFix/CytoPerm buffer is a fixation/permeabilization buffer containing formaldehyde and saponin for cell permeabilization. The BD Perm/Wash buffer is a saponin-containing wash buffer to aid in saponin-based permeabilization. It is particularly important that all steps of this protocol are performed using saponin-containing buffers.

Other intracellular molecules besides cytokines can also be assessed by flow cytometry. The protocols for these techniques are generally similar to those presented here with two changes: in vitro cell stimulation is not used and alcohol-based permeabilization methods are sometimes necessary. Specific protocols vary for individual signaling molecules and often require optimization.

13. Lympholyte M and other ficolls are sucrose solutions that allow for cell separation based on density. Lympholyte M should be stored at 4 °C to prevent contamination once it has been opened. Lympholyte M should be brought to room temperature before use to ensure that it is at the correct density when used to separate cells.

14. Cells at this stage can be stored for short periods of time at 4 °C or may be cryopreserved for later use. Cryopreservation may influence cell performance in functional assays.

15. Flow cytometry experiments require unstained cell controls and controls stained with each of the antibodies individually for setting voltages and compensation. We often stain compensation control beads instead of cells for our single-color controls (BD Biosciences). This allows conservation of cells and measurable staining with even those antibodies that stain rare populations. Unstained cells are still required to properly set up the flow cytometer. For complex experiments, we also use fluorescence minus one (FMO) gating controls. In an FMO control, all antibodies in a panel except for one are used to stain cells. This aids in setting negative gates [12].

16. We sometimes include MHC–peptide tetramers to allow for staining of antigen-specific T lymphocytes. If staining with tetramers, the protocol should be modified as follows:
    (a) Add an appropriate amount of tetramer to stain cells. Vortex all samples and incubate them for 30 min on ice in the dark.
    (b) Prepare a cocktail containing appropriate amounts of all of the surface-staining antibodies before staining and add this cocktail to the cells to stain. Add individual diluted antibodies to single-color control tubes. Vortex all samples and incubate them for 30 min on ice in the dark.

    Tetramers should always be added before antibodies, particularly anti-CD3, to allow tetramer access to TCR without hindrance from other antibodies. Antibodies against T cell variable regions sometimes require the same protocol modifications.

17. **Steps 4–6** are optional and are only necessary if you are interested in staining for surface antigens in addition to intracellular

antigens. The concentrations listed on the data sheets included with antibodies are often a useful place to start for initial staining experiments. Antibodies can usually be diluted further than suggested on the data sheets and careful titration can save on reagents and allow for cleaner staining.

18. CFSE is a cell-permeable dye that labels proteins. Staining must be performed in serum-free media to ensure that cellular proteins and not serum proteins are labeled. Once staining is complete, the cells should be washed with a large volume of media containing serum to quench the staining reaction. We have used different types of media (HBSS, PBS, RPMI) for the staining reaction with no adverse effects as long as the staining was in a serum-free media and the wash was in a serum-containing media.
19. The CFSE staining protocol listed utilizes large number of cells. It is also possible to stain smaller number of cells with protocol modifications, including adding serum to the staining reaction. This helps the cells survive the toxicity associated with CFSE staining. Vortexing should be avoided during CFSE staining to aid in cell viability.
20. Stimulation of all T cells in a mixed population can be achieved with azide-free anti-CD3 antibody or a mixture of PMA/ionomycin. PMA/ionomycin is preferred for short-term cytokine production, but does result in substantial cell death. Anti-CD3 is preferred for proliferation of cells in culture, but must be azide free to allow cells to proliferate. These reagents are useful positive controls to determine the maximum capacity of your cells to produce cytokines or proliferate as compared to cells stimulated with a specific antigen. Unstimulated cells are also important negative controls. Stimulation is not necessary when directly measuring cytokine production ex vivo and stimulation steps may be excluded in these cases.
21. Rat IL-2 allows for optimal T cell survival in culture.
22. Intracellular cytokine staining is a lengthy procedure. We have had good luck with the following modifications in order to spread the procedure over 2 days: (**a**) utilizing a heat block on a timer to incubate **step 3** at 37 °C for 6 h followed by cooling to 4 °C until the next day or manually moving cells to 4 °C following the 6-h incubation, and (**b**) incubating **step 7** at 4 °C overnight.
23. While using multichannel plates and plate washers makes the ELISPOT protocol less laborious, they can also create problems with the protocol. Be sure not to touch the membrane with your pipette tips or the plate washer. Multiscreen plates are generally quite sensitive and should be treated with care.

References

1. Eisenbarth SC, Williams A, Colegio OR, Meng H, Strowig T, Rongvaux A, Henao-Mejia J, Thaiss CA, Joly S, Gonzalez DG, Xu L, Zenewicz LA, Haberman AM, Elinav E, Kleinstein SH, Sutterwala FS, Flavell RA (2012) NLRP10 is a NOD-like receptor essential to initiate adaptive immunity by dendritic cells. Nature 484:510–513
2. Ippagunta SK, Malireddi RK, Shaw PJ, Neale GA, Walle LV, Green DR, Fukui Y, Lamkanfi M, Kanneganti TD (2011) The inflammasome adaptor ASC regulates the function of adaptive immune cells by controlling Dock2-mediated Rac activation and actin polymerization. Nat Immunol 12:1010–1016
3. Arthur JC, Lich JD, Ye Z, Allen IC, Gris D, Wilson JE, Schneider M, Roney KE, O'Connor BP, Moore CB, Morrison A, Sutterwala FS, Bertin J, Koller BH, Liu Z, Ting JP (2010) Cutting edge: NLRP12 controls dendritic and myeloid cell migration to affect contact hypersensitivity. J Immunol 185:4515–4519
4. Ichinohe T, Lee HK, Ogura Y, Flavell R, Iwasaki A (2009) Inflammasome recognition of influenza virus is essential for adaptive immune responses. J Exp Med 206:79–87
5. Mills KH (2011) TLR-dependent T cell activation in autoimmunity. Nat Rev Immunol 11:807–822
6. Manicassamy S, Pulendran B (2009) Modulation of adaptive immunity with toll-like receptors. Semin Immunol 21:185–193
7. Kronenberg M, Kinjo Y (2009) Innate-like recognition of microbes by invariant natural killer cells. Curr Opin Immunol 21:391–396
8. Sun JC, Lanier LL (2011) NK cell development, homeostasis, and function: parallels with CD8+ T cells. Nat Rev Immunol 11:645–657
9. Godfrey DI, Rossjohn J (2011) New ways to turn on NKT cells. J Exp Med 208:1121–1125
10. Born WK, Jin N, Aydintug MK, Wands JM, French JD, Roark CL, O'Brien RL (2007) gammadelta T lymphocytes-selectable cells within the innate system. J Clin Immunol 27:133–144
11. Krutzik PO, Irish JM, Nolan GP, Perez OD (2004) Analysis of protein phosphorylation and cellular signaling events by flow cytometry: techniques and clinical applications. Clin Immunol 110:206–221
12. Roederer M (2002) Compensation in flow cytometry. Curr Protocols Cytometry. Chapter 1 Unit 1.4

Chapter 11

Bioassay for the Measurement of Type-I Interferon Activity

Douglas G. Widman

Abstract

Type I interferons are critical cytokines produced by the host innate immune response to viral infection. They act collectively to initiate expression of a multitude of antiviral genes that serve to inhibit viral replication and spread. Despite the great importance of interferons to the host response to viral infection, assays to measure their presence can be costly and require a great deal of optimization for success. Here, we describe an inexpensive approach for the determination of murine type I interferon activity in a given set of samples, which is based on using 50 % protection of a cell monolayer from virus-induced cytopathic effects as an endpoint measurement. The following protocol allows for the accurate and sensitive measurement of interferon activity without the use of highly specialized equipment or reagents.

Key words Interferon, Type I, Interferon alpha, Interferon beta, Encephalomyocarditis virus, EMCV, Innate immunity, Virus

1 Introduction

Since their discovery in 1957, type I interferons (IFN) have been widely appreciated as the key mediators of antiviral innate immune responses [1]. They work in both autocrine and paracrine fashions to initiate the expression of a wide array of genes that serve to create an antiviral state in host cells, which serves to suppress viral replication and spread. A number of assays exist for the measurement of IFN in a set of samples including enzyme-linked immunosorbent assay (ELISA), intracellular cytokine staining, and western blot. The primary disadvantage of these assays is that they depend on IFN-specific antibodies for their success, and heretofore these antibodies have been expensive and require a great deal of optimization for effective use. However, the IFN bioassay described here is relatively inexpensive and straightforward to perform. It provides a functional readout of IFN activity by measuring the ability of a given sample to protect L929 cells against encephalomyocarditis virus (EMCV)-mediated cytopathic effect (CPE). The protocol is highly

Irving C. Allen (ed.), *Mouse Models of Innate Immunity: Methods and Protocols*, Methods in Molecular Biology, vol. 1031, DOI 10.1007/978-1-62703-481-4_11, © Springer Science+Business Media, LLC 2013

flexible and requires little optimization to obtain useful results. A number of variations to this protocol have been developed and are frequently utilized, including modifications to cell type (murine, human, or bovine fibroblasts) and challenge virus (vesicular stomatitis virus or Semliki Forest virus). One major advantage of this protocol over many others is the ability to distinguish between the antiviral activity of type I interferons (IFNα/β) and type II interferon (IFNγ). Overnight acidification of the samples to a pH of 2–3 destroys any IFNγ in the samples while preserving IFNα/β activity. This allows for the specific IFNα/β antiviral activity to be measured. The total time required to complete this assay is 4 days, so careful preplanning is recommended.

2 Materials

2.1 Cell Line and Virus

1. L929 mouse fibroblast cells (American Type Culture Collection).
2. EMCV (American Type Culture Collection) (*see* **Note 1**).

2.2 Media and Solutions

1. Sterile distilled water.
2. 1× Phosphate-buffered saline (PBS).
3. Eagle's minimum essential medium (MEM).
4. Fetal bovine serum (FBS) (*see* **Note 2**).
5. Nonessential amino acids (NEAA) (10 mM).
6. Streptomycin (10,000 μg) and penicillin (10,000 U) solution.
7. L-Glutamine solution (200 mM).
8. Sodium pyruvate solution (100 mM).
9. Trypsin–EDTA (0.05 %).
10. Growth medium: MEM containing 10 % FBS, 1 % L-glutamine, 1 % NEAA, 1 % sodium pyruvate, and 1 % pen/strep solution.
11. Isopropanol (2-propanol).
12. 2 N HCl (0.2 μm filter sterilized).
13. 2 N NaOH (prepared in sterile water).
14. 0.04 N HCl in isopropanol.
15. Thiazolyl blue tetrazolium bromide (also known as methylthiazolyldiphenyl-tetrazolium bromide; MTT) (*see* **Note 3**).
16. Mouse IFN beta standard (*see* **Note 4**).

2.3 Tissue Culture Plastics, Materials, and Equipment

1. Flat-bottom 96-well tissue culture-treated plates.
2. Litmus paper.
3. 12-well multichannel pipette (20–200 μl) with tips.

4. Inverted microscope (with 10× and 20× objectives).
5. Hemacytometer.
6. Handheld 254 nm wavelength ultraviolet lamp.

3 Methods

3.1 L929 Cell Preparation (See Note 5)

1. Cultivate L929 cells at 37 °C and 5 % CO_2 with subcultivation at a ratio of 1:4 to 1:6 approximately twice weekly. Remove the growth medium from L929 cells growing in large flasks or tissue culture dishes and rinse once with 1× PBS.
2. Add enough trypsin to coat the cell monolayer (1–2 ml), and incubate at 37 °C for 60–90 s. Verify that the majority of the cells are no longer attached to the plate by observing under a 10× inverted microscope and tapping gently.
3. Once cells are detached, resuspend cells in a total volume of 10–20 ml of growth medium.
4. Count live cells under a 20× inverted microscope using a hemacytometer.
5. Resuspend the quantified L929 cells to a concentration of 3.0×10^5 cells per ml.
6. Using a multichannel pipette, add 100 μl of L929 cell suspension to each well of a 96-well plate to achieve 3.0×10^4 cells per well.
7. Place plates in a 37 °C and 5 % CO_2 incubator overnight.

3.2 Preparation of Standards and Unknown Samples

1. Dilute unknown samples in L929 medium. For mock-treated samples, dilute 1:2–1:4. For virus-infected samples, dilute 1:8–1:10 (*see* **Note 6**). The final diluted volume should be 300 μl, at minimum.
2. Prepare the IFN beta standard by diluting the stock to a concentration of 1,000 U/ml in L929 medium (*see* **Note 7**).
3. Acidify all unknown samples and standards with 2 N HCl to pH = 2–3. Pipette a few drops onto litmus paper to verify the pH. Incubate the samples for 20–24 h at 4 °C.

3.3 Addition of Standards and Unknowns to Cell Monolayers

1. Neutralize the samples and standards to pH = 7.4 with 2 N NaOH. Pipette a few drops onto litmus paper to verify the pH. Set the samples aside on ice. Neutralization to pH = 7.4 is critical for cell viability throughout the rest of this assay as these samples will be applied directly to L929 cells.
2. UV inactivate residual virus in unknown samples by transferring 300 μl of each unknown sample into a 48-well plate and place on ice 5–6 cm from the UV source. Expose the plate to UV radiation for 10 min.

3. Prepare the 96-well plates containing L929 cells for the addition of samples and standards. Typically, 6 wells of row A are reserved for positive and negative (+virus and –virus) controls, respectively. Row B is used for standards, and rows C–H for unknown samples (two rows for each). Serial dilutions of samples and standards are made from left to right across the plate.
4. Add 100 μl of neutralized (pH = 7.4) IFN beta standard to the first well of the standards row on each of the 96-well plates containing L929 cells. This is typically well B1. Add 100 μl of each unknown sample to the first wells of two rows on the 96-well plates. For example, unknown #1 will be added to wells C1 and D1, unknown #2 will be added to wells E1 and F1, and continuing through the rest of the plate for each sample. Do not remove the medium from the plates prior to the addition of standard and samples. The first well of each row will be a 1:2 dilution of the neutralized samples/standards. Using a multichannel pipette, make two-fold serial dilutions by transferring 100 μl from the first well to adjacent wells. Discard 100 μl from the final dilution row so that all wells contain 100 μl. Do not add anything to +virus and –virus wells in row A. Incubate the plate for 24 h at 37 °C and 5 % CO_2.

3.4 Inoculation of Cells with EMCV Challenge Virus

1. Prepare the EMCV challenge virus by diluting the virus stock to 4×10^6 pfu/ml in L929 medium. Add 50 μl/well to all wells except the –virus wells. Do not remove medium from any wells prior to the addition of virus. Incubate the plates for 18–24 h at 37 °C and 5 % CO_2.

3.5 MTT Cell Viability Assay and Data Collection

1. Prepare the MTT (*see* **Note 3**) by preparing a solution of 6 mg/ml of MTT in L929 medium. Each plate requires 1.5 ml of this solution.
2. Using a multichannel pipette, add 15 μl of MTT to each well and incubate for 2–4 h at 37 °C and 5 % CO_2.
3. Aspirate MTT-containing supernatant from all wells into a hazardous waste bottle (*see* **Note 3**).
4. Add 100 μl/well of 0.04 N HCl in isopropanol to all wells.
5. Incubate the plate at room temperature for 10–15 min.
6. Add 100 μl/well of distilled water.
7. Analyze the absorbance of each well on a 96-well-based optical plate reader at 570 nm wavelength.

3.6 Analysis of Bioassay Data

1. Determine the optical density (OD) for the 50 % lethal dose of EMCV (LD_{50}) by calculating the total average of the 6 +virus wells and the 6 –virus wells.
2. Determine the 2 wells in the IFN standard row that are closest to the LD_{50} OD. These will be used to back calculate the starting

concentration of the IFN standard. Use the formula $x = (2^y) \times z$: where x is the starting concentration of the IFN standard on the plate (usually 500 U/ml); y is the average of the 2 wells between which the LD_{50} OD falls (*see* **Note 8**); and z is the average concentration of the IFN standard between the 2 determined wells (*see* **Note 9**). Because the LD_{50} OD will not always equal the median of the OD of the 2 wells in the standard dilution curve, it may be necessary to modify the z value in order to make x equal the known starting concentration of the IFN standard (*see* **Note 10**). This is critical in determining the concentrations of the unknown samples, as this z value will be used for all subsequent calculations.

3. Repeat **step 2** for each of the unknown samples. First determine the value for y for each unknown (*see* **Note 8**), and then plug that value into the equation $x = (2^y) \times z$: where z is the value determined in **step 2**. x will be the IFN concentration of the sample as it was loaded onto the plate. Multiply this value by any dilution factor applied to the samples before they were added to the plate. Calculate the average of the duplicate results, and report IFN activity in U/ml.

4 Notes

1. EMCV is infectious and is classified as a BSL-2 pathogen. Materials in this category present a moderate risk to laboratory personnel and should be handled under standard BSL-2 guidelines. Additional pathogen-specific institutional, local, and national regulatory guidelines apply. All infectious materials should be handled under the direct supervision of competent and knowledgeable laboratory personnel. A material transfer agreement (MTA) with ATCC is required for the use of this pathogen.
2. This protocol has been optimized for the use of heat-inactivated (56 °C for 30 min) FBS. It is possible that non-heat-inactivated FBS may be used; however, some optimization may be required.
3. MTT is classified as an irritant and mutagen. It is capable of causing skin (category 2) and eye (category 2A) irritation as well as germ cell mutagenicity (category 2) and specific target organ toxicity from a single dose (category 3). Care should be taken when preparing solutions and handling waste. Personal protective equipment should be utilized to prevent contact with skin, airways, and mucous membranes. All solutions containing MTT along with equipment (tips, tubes, weigh boats, etc.) that comes into contact with MTT should be disposed of using approved hazardous waste disposal protocols. Additional hazardous material-specific institutional, local, and

national regulatory guidelines apply. Consult MSDS for further information.

4. The IFN standard should be divided into small single-use aliquots and stored at −80 °C. It is not recommended reusing previously thawed aliquots, and a fresh standard should be used each time the assay is run.
5. It is important to determine the number of 96-well plates that will be necessary to assay the unknown samples. Generally, plates are set up using 2 horizontal rows (samples are run in duplicate) of a 96-well plate for each unknown. One horizontal row at minimum must also be reserved for the IFN beta standard (this can optionally be run in duplicate), and one row is reserved for positive and negative controls (+virus and −virus). Therefore, 3 unknown samples can be assayed on a single 96-well plate when a single row of standard is used.
6. This is only a guide and careful empirical determination of appropriate dilutions should be made for a given set of samples.
7. This is only a guide and careful empirical determination of the IFN beta concentrations necessary to produce a standard curve within which the concentrations of the unknown samples fall is recommended.
8. For example, if the LD_{50} OD falls between wells B6 and B7 on the row of IFN standard, then $y = 6.5$. Note that this is the average of the well numbers on the plate, and not the OD values of the wells.
9. For example, if starting IFN concentration is 500 U/ml in well B1, and the LD_{50} OD falls between wells B6 and B7, $z = 11.72$.
10. 500 U/ml in this case.

Reference

1. Isaacs A, Lindenmann J (1957) Virus interference. I. The interferon. Proc R Soc Lond B Biol Sci 147(927):258–267

Chapter 12

Safe and Effective Mouse Footpad Inoculation

Kristin M. Long and Mark Heise

Abstract

Footpad injection is an important route of inoculation in mouse models of disease and immunology. Although commonly used to deliver antigens as a means of eliciting an efficacious immunological response, herein, we describe a protocol for inoculating mice via footpad injection using a hands-free method to deliver infectious material. These procedures allow for efficient delivery of infectious agents in a manner that is safe for both the researcher and animal.

Key words Footpad, Viral inoculation, Arbovirus, Mouse, Hands-free inoculation

1 Introduction

Footpad inoculation provides for a combination of intradermal and subcutaneous injection in the mouse model. It has primarily been used as a route of vaccination, and for the administration of certain neurotracer dyes. It has been a popular method for immunological studies because the path of draining lymph from the footpad is well characterized and provides three lymph node locations for analysis of immunological response: popliteal [1], sub-iliac [2], and inguinal [3]. In addition to vaccines and chemicals, footpad inoculation has been a useful tool in the study of viruses including members of the Flaviviridae, Poxviridae, and Togaviridae families. The ability to infect a host through a breach in the epidermis and dermis, such as what may occur through the bite of an infected insect vector, is a common feature of viruses in these families. There are several factors which make the inoculation of pathogens using the footpad method more elaborate than introducing antigens using the same route. Notably, the small area of the mouse footpad coupled with the use of sharps to deliver infectious virus raises concerns regarding researcher safety. Therefore, we have developed a hands-free inoculation system for footpad infection of mice that keeps the hands of the researcher clear of the site of inoculation with the option of lightly anesthetizing the mouse.

Irving C. Allen (ed.), *Mouse Models of Innate Immunity: Methods and Protocols*, Methods in Molecular Biology, vol. 1031, DOI 10.1007/978-1-62703-481-4_12,

2 Materials

2.1 Virus Preparation

1. Prepare virus of interest following a standard protocol.
2. Prepare inoculum such that each mouse will receive a 0.01 ml dose of virus. Although some protocols allow for 0.05 ml of inoculum, we have found that 0.01 ml of inoculum is an ideal volume for mice of any age. As the volume of inoculum increases, so does the risk of leakage of the virus once the needle is removed from the injection site.

2.2 Equipment

1. Hamilton 100 μL, model 710 leur tip syringe.
2. 30 gauge ½ in. needles.
3. Inhalation anesthesia, such as isoflurane.
4. Jar for anesthesia, such as a Wheaton clear glass 16 oz straight sided jar with screw cap.
5. Cotton pads or batting.
6. Aluminum foil.
7. Straight, cover glass forceps.
8. Broome style rodent restrainer.

3 Methods

1. If using anesthesia, prepare the drop jar. A capful of isoflurane is added to cotton and placed in the bottom of the jar. A piece of aluminum foil is then added over the cotton to keep the mouse from coming in direct contact with the anesthetic.
2. Hamilton syringes must be primed before use. The tip of a sterilized syringe should be placed into the inoculum and the plunger pulled back to the marking for 0.1 ml. The syringe is then removed from the liquid and a capped needle is firmly attached to the syringe. Inverting the syringe, remove the cap and slowly depress the plunger until a small drop of liquid appears at the end of the needle. This indicates that all air has been removed from the needle.
3. Reinsert the needle back into the tube of inoculum and fill the syringe to the proper marking **Note 5**. It is left to the discretion of the researcher whether they load multiple doses or a single dose.
4. Lightly anesthetize the mouse using drop method anesthesia, unless anesthesia is contraindicated for the particular experiment.
5. Remove the mouse from the jar and insert into a Broome restrainer by grasping the foot to be inoculated (**Note 1**) and pull the foot through the slot to the outside of the restrainer.

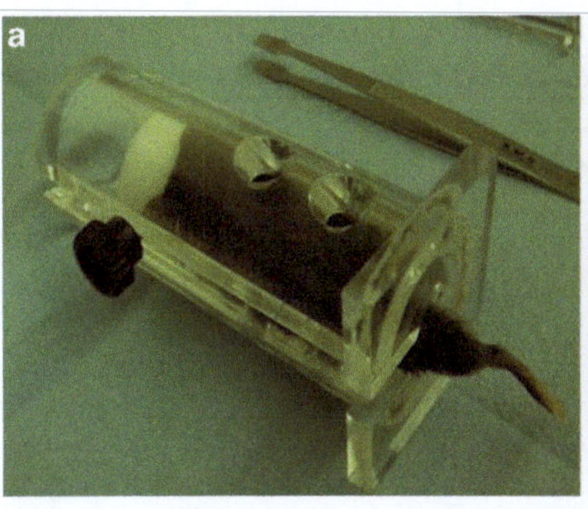

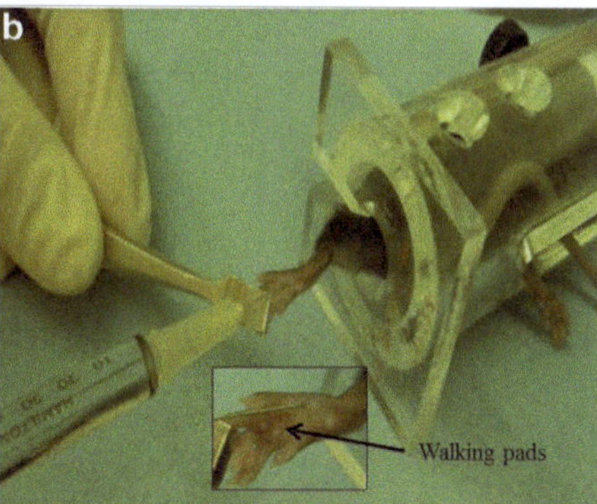

Fig. 1 Illustration demonstrating the proper restraint of the mouse for hands-free footpad inoculation. (**a**) Following light anesthesia, the mouse is pulled through the restrainer by the foot to be inoculated so that the foot is brought to the outside of the restrainer and the mouse is secured. (**b**) The foot is then grasped lightly with flat forceps and a 30 gauge ½ in. needle attached to a Hamilton syringe is used to administer the inoculum subcutaneously into the footpad directly between the ankle and walking pads (*inset*). Allow 3–5 s before removing the needle to allow the inoculum time to disperse to minimize leakage from the inoculation site

Ensure that the ventral side of the foot faces upwards. Secure the mouse in the restrainer (Fig. 1a).

6. Grasp the foot just above the toes with the forceps. Lay the needle on top of the foot with the bevel side up and insert the needle just under the skin between the walking pads and the heel **Note 3** (Fig. 1b).
7. Deliver the inoculum and wait 3–5 s after delivery before slowly removing the needle. This will minimize fluid leakage from the injection site **Note 4**. Release the foot with the forceps and return the mouse to the cage **Note 2**.

4 Notes

1. All works involving animals and infectious agents are performed in accordance with guidelines and approval from animal care and use committees and biological safety regulations. Since mice use their forefeet for handling food, animal care and use regulations generally prohibit the use of the forefeet for footpad injections. In addition, regulations may also limit inoculations to only one hind foot per animal.
2. Mice that are awake may be aggressive when coming out of the restrainer. Use proper animal handling techniques to minimize the possibility of a bite.
3. If the inoculation draws blood, the puncture went beyond the dermal layer and the researcher should make note as the introduction of virus into the bloodstream may skew results.
4. Leakage may occur if the needle is withdrawn too quickly and inoculum is not allowed to disperse before the needle is removed.

5. Due to the small volume of inoculum, ensure accuracy by following the manufacturer's instructions for measuring in a Hamilton syringe.

References

1. Kawashim Y, Sugimura M, Hwang Y et al (1964) Lymph system in mice. Jpn J Vet Res 12:69–72
2. Van den Broeck W, Derore A, Simoens P (2006) Anatomy and nomenclature of murine lymph nodes: descriptive study and nomenclatory standardization in BALB/cAnNCrl mice. J Immunol Meth 312(1–2):12–19
3. Tilney N (1971) Patterns of lymphatic drainage in the adult laboratory rat. J Anat 109(Pt 3): 369–383

Chapter 13

Delayed-Type Hypersensitivity Models in Mice

Irving C. Allen

Abstract

Delayed-type hypersensitivity (DTH) is a useful approach for evaluating cell-mediated immune responses associated with Th1 reactivity. The DTH reaction is divided into the afferent and efferent phases. During the afferent phase of this model, mice are typically immunized by subcutaneous injection with a specific hapten or antigen in its chemically reactive state and emulsified with an adjuvant. The efferent phase is typically initiated 5–12 days after sensitization, whereby the previously sensitized mice are challenged by either subcutaneous footpad injection or intradermal ear injection. The DTH response is evaluated 24 h post challenge. Here, we describe a common protocol for the induction and assessment of the DTH reaction in mice using keyhole limpet hemocyanin.

Key words CHS, Contact hypersensitivity, DTH, Intradermal injection, In vivo, Keyhole limpet hemocyanin, KLH, Th1, Th2

1 Introduction

The delayed-type hypersensitivity (DTH) reaction is a prototypical in vivo assay to study cell-mediated host immune function. The DTH reaction is mediated by CD4+ T lymphocytes, which promote T-helper cell type 1 (Th1) production of interferon-γ. The inflammatory reaction to antigen typically peaks within 48 h post exposure. In humans, there are two common forms of DTH reactions, the tuberculin DTH reaction and contact sensitivity. The tuberculin DTH reaction is a cell-mediated reaction following subcutaneous injection with bacterial or viral antigens, whereas the contact sensitivity reaction is associated with epicutaneous exposure in sensitized individuals. In both humans and mice, the DTH reaction consists of two distinct stages, the afferent/sensitization phase and the efferent/elicitation phase. In mouse models, during the sensitization phase, animals are subcutaneously exposed to a specific protein or hapten allergen that is typically emulsified with an adjuvant. Following exposure, dendritic cells and Langerhans cells from the deposition site traffic

Irving C. Allen (ed.), *Mouse Models of Innate Immunity: Methods and Protocols*, Methods in Molecular Biology, vol. 1031, DOI 10.1007/978-1-62703-481-4_13, © Springer Science+Business Media, LLC 2013

from the epidermal layers to the draining lymph nodes, where they present antigen-major histocompatibility complex (MHC) entities to T lymphocytes [1–4]. During the elicitation phase, animals are reexposed to the allergen used for sensitization by either dermal injection into the ear pinna or by paw-pad injection, which results in the trafficking of allergen-specific T lymphocytes to the site of antigen deposition and the subsequent production of proinflammatory cytokines [4]. The DTH response can be evaluated by assessments of localized swelling, leukocyte infiltration of the challenged tissues, and Th1-associated cytokine profiling. In this chapter, we describe the detailed protocols for the induction and evaluation of the DTH reaction in mice.

2 Materials

2.1 Mice

1. Adult female (*see* **Note 1**) 6–8-week-old Balb/c mice (*see* **Note 2**) that have been bred (*see* **Note 3**) and housed under specific pathogen-free conditions (*see* **Note 4**).
2. Mice should be acclimated to the housing facility for at least 5 days prior to the beginning of the experiment.

2.2 Reagents and Solutions

1. 70 % Ethanol (EtOH).
2. Keyhole limpet hemocyanin (KLH) (*see* **Note 5**).
3. Incomplete Freund's adjuvant (IFA).
4. Complete Freund's adjuvant (CFA).
5. 1× Phosphate-buffered saline (PBS).
6. 10 % Neutral buffered formalin.
7. Avertin: 2,2,2 Tribromoethanol and amylene hydrate (*see* **Note 6**).
8. Isoflurane.

2.3 Materials and Equipment

1. Tissue homogenizer.
2. 10 or 25 μl Hamilton Syringe.
3. 1 ml syringe (27 g needle).
4. Forceps.
5. Scissors.
6. 8 mm leather hole punch.
7. Cork board.
8. Analytical balance.
9. Calipers (dial thickness gauge 0.01–12.5 mm).
10. Indelible marking pen.
11. 24-Well tissue culture plates.
12. Round-bottom 5 or 10 ml tube.

3 Methods

3.1 Preparation of Emulsion by Mechanically Mixing (See Note 7) [5]

1. Determine the required volumes of KLH, IFA, and CFA in a 1:1:1 ratio to make the emulsion. The animals will receive injections totaling 100 μl of the emulsion during the sensitization phase. Each animal will receive 100 μg of KLH. The minimum amount of KLH and adjuvant that can be emulsified using this protocol is 500 μl and calculations should include an additional 300 μl to adjust for loss of material.
2. Using a tissue homogenizer, gently mix the IFA and CFA in the round-bottom tube. While mixing, slowly add the KLH. Once the KLH has been added, increase the speed of the homogenizer to maximum speed for approximately 2 min. It is *critical* that the mixture remain on ice throughout the entire emulsification process.
3. Visually inspect the emulsion to ensure that it is thoroughly mixed. The emulsion should have the appearance and viscosity of dense whipped cream [5]. Continue to mix the emulsion until the emulsification is satisfactory.

3.2 Delayed-Type Hypersensitivity (Sensitization)

1. Anesthetize mice using drop method isoflurane (*see* **Note 8**).
2. Sensitize the mice by subcutaneous injection of freshly prepared KLH (100 μg) emulsified in IFA and CFA [6, 7]. Mice should be injected with 50 μl of the KLH emulsion in two different locations between the shoulder blades. The injection sites should be cleaned with ethanol, but not shaven to avoid possible skin damage or additional irritation.

3.3 Delayed-Type Hypersensitivity (Ear Pinna Elicitation)

1. The elicitation phase should be evaluated between 5 and 12 days after sensitization.
2. Prepare KLH solution in sterile pyrogen-free saline for intradermal ear pinna injection. Each mouse will receive an injection of 10 μg of KLH in 10 μl of PBS into the right pinna and 10 μl of PBS vehicle alone into the left pinna [6, 7].
3. Mice should be anesthetized using freshly prepared avertin, following all required institutional policies and regulations.
4. Measure baseline pinna thickness for both ears using calipers (*see* **Note 9**).
5. Immediately following pinna thickness assessments, using a hamilton syringe, intradermally inject 10 μl of the KLH solution into the right ear (KLH challenged) and 10 μl of PBS into the left ear (vehicle control) (*see* **Note 10**). Additional controls should also include mice that were sensitized, but received PBS injections in both pinna and mice that were challenged in the

pinna, but never sensitized. Naïve mice should also be included for reference (*see* **Note 11**).

6. Identify each animal using tail marks with the indelible pen for temporary identification.

3.4 Pinna Harvest

1. Twenty-four hours post elicitation, measure pinna thickness using calipers.
2. Calculate the change in pinna thickness (ΔT) using the following equation:

$$\Delta T = (\text{pinna thickness 24 h following elicitation}) - (\text{baseline pinna thickness})$$

Calculate ΔT for both the right (KLH challenged) pinna and left (unchallenged) pinna and show as either ΔT or percent change.

3. Euthanize the mice following appropriate institutional guidelines (*see* **Note 4**).
4. Optional: If systemic assessments of circulating cytokines or immunoglobulins are desired, whole blood can be collected utilizing cardiac puncture immediately following euthanasia for serum evaluation.
5. Remove the left and right pinna, taking care to keep the KLH-treated and vehicle control ears separate (*see* **Note 12**).
6. Once all of the pinna are removed from the mice, place each individual pinna on a cork board and use the 8 mm leather punch to remove the central most portion of the pinna. The punch should include the majority of the pinna and be located in the same area for all animals, taking care to avoid the thicker cartilage at the base.
7. Weigh each 8 mm pinna punch using an analytical scale.
8. Calculate the change in pinna weight (ΔW) between the KLH-challenged pinna and the unchallenged pinna using the following equation:

$$\Delta W = (\text{pinna weight of the hapten challenged ear}) - (\text{pinna weight of the vehicle treated ear})$$

Show as either ΔW or percent change.

9. Following weight assessments, each pinna punch should be fixed in 10 % neutral buffered formalin, paraffin embedded, sectioned, and H&E stained for histology (*see* **Note 13**). Immune cell infiltration and histopathology can then be evaluated [8].

4 Notes

1. Female mice are preferred in these assays due to their more docile nature. There is an increased probability that adult male animals will become aggressive during the course of this type of experiment, which can lead to fight wounds and ear damage. If male mice are to be utilized, consider individual housing.
2. We have successfully utilized 6–12-week-old C57Bl/6, 129SvEv, and BALB/c mice in these assays. If strain is not a limiting factor, BALB/c mice are preferred due to their robust response in the ear swelling assays. It is possible that some aspects of this protocol may need to be adjusted and further optimized when using mice from different genetic backgrounds.
3. When breeding and identifying mice by ear punch or ear tag, all attempts should be made to limit excessive damage to the ears and preserve the tissue integrity. If possible, avoid using ear punch or ear tags to identify mice directed to DTH studies.
4. All studies should be conducted in accordance with the local and institutional animal care and use guidelines and in accordance with the prevailing national regulations.
5. KLH is used in the following protocol. However, other common antigens have been successfully used to instigate the DTH reaction including ovalbumin, Np-O-Su, bacille Calmette–Guérin (BCG), various haptens, and microbial constituents. The experimental conditions described here will require optimization prior to the utilization of other antigens. Typical elements requiring modification include the choice of adjuvant, the location of the sensitization (i.e., shoulder, belly, or base of tail), mouse strain, and location of elicitation (i.e., footpad or pinna).
6. Avertin is the trademark name for tribromoethanol. Most institutions have strict guidelines regarding the preparation and use of tribromoethanol as an anesthetic. Tribromoethanol should always be prepared fresh before each use and each mouse should only receive a single intraperitoneal injection. Avertin-induced anesthesia requires 1–2 min and is effective for approximately 40–90 min.
7. There are many protocols for generating emulsions. The mechanical protocol described here is rapid and produces a high-quality emulsion. However, a major limitation of this method is the generation of heat, which may result in protein denaturing. Therefore, it is essential that the emulsion be maintained on ice throughout the emulsification procedure. Depending on the specific antigen, this method may be suboptimal and a manual method of emulsification should be considered. Mechanical emulsification should always be done under a hood or preferably in a biological safety cabinet to limit exposure to aerosols.

8. Drop method isoflurane induces a low level of anesthesia that is recommended for this procedure, but is not necessary. We have found that light anesthesia allows for more accurate subcutaneous injections in the animals and reduces variability in this assay. This method induces anesthesia within 30 s and will lightly anesthetize the mouse for approximately 30 s. Each individual institution will have specific guidelines regarding the use of drop method anesthesia.
9. The caliper assessments of ear thickness are the most likely source of error in this procedure. Thus, it is essential that individuals be trained and practice using calipers to assess ear thickness prior to the start of this procedure. As an alternative to calipers or to confirm the caliper findings, ear thickness can be assessed using digital imaging [8].
10. One of the strengths of this model is the ability to evaluate the DTH reaction using experimental and control ears from the same animal.
11. In general, there will be a high level of variability in this model due to the complex nature of the DTH response. Therefore, large groups of mice should be used. We typically prefer >7 animals per group. Likewise, the health and age of the animals can dramatically influence the DTH response.
12. We have found that placing the pinna in individual wells in a labeled 24-well tissue culture plate is ideal.
13. As an alternative to histology evaluation, the 8 mm pinna punches can also be frozen on dry ice or by liquid nitrogen and manually homogenized for protein or RNA extraction using standard protocols and reagents.

References

1. Hemmi H, Yoshino M, Yamazaki H, Naito M, Iyoda T, Omatsu Y, Shimoyama S, Letterio JJ, Nakabayashi T, Tagaya H, Yamane T, Ogawa M, Nishikawa S, Ryoke K, Inaba K, Hayashi S, Kunisada T (2001) Skin antigens in the steady state are trafficked to regional lymph nodes by transforming growth factor-beta1-dependent cells. Int Immunol 13:695–704
2. Yoshino M, Yamazaki H, Nakano H, Kakiuchi T, Ryoke K, Kunisada T, Hayashi S (2003) Distinct antigen trafficking from skin in the steady and active states. Int Immunol 15: 773–779
3. Yoshino M, Yamazaki H, Shultz LD, Hayashi S (2006) Constant rate of steady-state self antigen trafficking from skin to regional lymph nodes. Int Immunol 18:1541–1548
4. Dieli F, Sireci G, Salerno A, Bellavia A (1999) Impaired contact hypersensitivity to trinitrochlorobenzene in interleukin-4-deficient mice. Immunology 98:71–79
5. Brand DD, Latham KA, Rosloniec EF (2007) Collagen-induced arthritis. Nat Protocols 2(5):1269–1275
6. Engstrom L, Pinzon-Ortiz MC, Li Y, Chen S, Kinsley D, Nelissen R, Fine JS, Mihara K, Manfra D (2009) Characterization of a murine keyhole limpet hemocyanin (KLH)-delayed-type hypersensitivity (DTH) model: role for p38 kinase. Int Immunopharmacol 9: 1218–1227
7. Akahira-Azuma M, Szczepanik M, Tsuji RF, Campos RA, Itakura A, Mobini N, McNiff J, Kawikova I, Lu B, Gerard C, Jordan S (2004)

Early delayed-type hypersensitivity eosinophil infiltrates depend on T helper 2 cytokines and interferon-γ via CXCR3 chemokines. Immunology 111:306–317

8. Arthur JC, Lich JD, Ye Z, Allen IC, Gris D, Schneider M, Roney KE, O'Connor BP, Moore CB, Morrison A, Sutterwala FS, Koller BH, Bertin J, Liu Z, Ting JPY (2010) Cutting edge: NLRP12 controls dendritic and myeloid cell migration to affect contact hypersensitivity. J Immunol 185(8): 4515–4519

Chapter 14

Mouse Model of *Staphylococcus aureus* Skin Infection

Natalia Malachowa, Scott D. Kobayashi, Kevin R. Braughton, and Frank R. DeLeo

Abstract

Bacterial skin and soft tissue infections are abundant worldwide and many are caused by *Staphylococcus aureus*. Indeed, *S. aureus* is the leading cause of skin and soft tissue infections in the USA. Here, we describe a mouse model of skin and soft tissue infection induced by subcutaneous inoculation of *S. aureus*. This animal model can be used to investigate a number of factors related to the pathogenesis of skin and soft tissue infections, including strain virulence and the contribution of specific bacterial molecules to disease, and it can be employed to test the potential effectiveness of antibiotic therapies or vaccine candidates.

Key words Skin infection, Abscess, Bacteria, Mouse, *Staphylococcus aureus*

1 Introduction

Animal infection models are an integral part of host-pathogen research and are used to approximate the complex environment of the human body. Intact human skin is a unique and complex tissue that forms a physical barrier and serves as a frontline defense against invading microorganisms. In addition to functioning as a mechanical barrier, skin plays an essential role in both innate and adaptive immune defenses. For example, skin is comprised of numerous cell types including keratinocytes, Langerhans cells, and macrophages, which release immunomodulatory cytokines and chemokines that provide an early warning system during pathogen intrusion [1]. Moreover, professional phagocytes, such as recruited neutrophils and macrophages, are capable of ingesting and killing invading pathogens. Skin cells can also produce antimicrobial peptides, which provide an additional layer of defense against microbial pathogens [2]. Mechanically compromised skin and impaired skin function can lead to a wide range of dermatological diseases. Among these are inflammatory diseases such as atopic dermatitis and psoriasis, or skin cancers including melanomas. Nevertheless, the majority of skin diseases have an infectious etiology [3, 4]. Skin

Irving C. Allen (ed.), *Mouse Models of Innate Immunity: Methods and Protocols*, Methods in Molecular Biology, vol. 1031, DOI 10.1007/978-1-62703-481-4_14, © Springer Science+Business Media, LLC 2013

infections are caused by a taxonomic diversity of infectious microorganisms that include fungi, viruses [5], parasites [6–8], protozoa, and a variety of Gram-positive and Gram-negative bacterial species [9–11].

Staphylococcus aureus is one of the most prominent human pathogens and is a major cause of skin and soft tissue infections. In the USA, the community-associated methicillin-resistant *S. aureus* (CA-MRSA) strain USA300 is the predominant cause of skin and soft tissue infections [12–14]. The success of *S. aureus* as a human pathogen is dependent on several factors, including the ability to adapt to environmental changes and produce a variety of molecules that contribute to virulence. Several mouse models of infection have been developed to increase our understanding of staphylococcal pathogenesis [15–20]. In this chapter we describe a mouse model of *S. aureus* skin and soft tissue infection (SSTI) induced by subcutaneous inoculation of USA300. The methods described herein utilize commercially available reagents and can be reproduced by most standard laboratories.

2 Materials

These materials are for use with *S. aureus* as the infectious agent and can be altered to fit the culture requirements for any bacterium of interest.

2.1 Bacterial Culture and Inoculum

1. Trypticase Soy Broth (TSB) and Trypticase Soy Agar (TSA).
2. Sterile Dulbecco's phosphate-buffered saline (DPBS).
3. Sterile 3.5-mL clear screw cap septum vials.
4. *S. aureus* strain LAC (representative of the epidemic USA300 strain, NARSA # JE2, *see* **Note 1**).

2.2 Preparation of Mouse Skin for Infection

1. Xenogen XGI-8 Gas Anesthesia System with Matrix VIP3000 isoflurane vaporizer (Caliper Life Science, Hopkinton, MA).
2. Isoflurane.
3. Crl:SKH1-E outbred, immunocompetent, hairless or Balb/c female mice 6–8 weeks old, 20–25 g (Charles River Laboratories International, Inc., Wilmington, MA) (*see* **Note 2**).
4. Mice are housed in large (5 animals/cage) or small (3 animals/cage) cages and are allowed food and water ad libitum.
5. Finisher® electric trimmer with narrow blade (Oster® Direct, McMinnville, TN).
6. Nair® hair remover lotion (Church & Dwight Co. Inc., Princeton, NJ).
7. Gauze sponges, 3″ × 3″.

2.3 Subcutaneous Inoculation of Bacteria and Analysis of Skin Lesions

1. Scout™ ProSP202 scale (Ohaus Corporation, Pine Brook, NJ).
2. 1-mL syringe with tuberculin slip tip.
3. 27-G × ½ in. needles.
4. Digital calipers.

3 Methods

3.1 Preparation of Bacterial Inoculum

1. Inoculate *S. aureus* (from a frozen glycerol stock) into sterilized TSB media in a flask-to-media volume ratio of 5:1.
2. Grow the bacteria at 37 °C with rotary shaking (225 rpm) for 16–18 h (late stationary-phase of growth, OD_{600} ~2.1).
3. Transfer bacteria from late stationary-phase culture to fresh TSB media (1:200 dilution) and incubate at 37 °C with rotary shaking (225 rpm) until the optical density at 600 nm (OD_{600}) of the culture reaches 0.75 (~2–2.5 h for USA300, which is mid-exponential phase of growth) (*see* **Note 3**).
4. Collect bacteria by centrifugation (3,000 × *g*, 4 °C for 10 min). Bacteria are maintained at ~4 °C until ready for inoculation by incubation on ice (*see* **Note 4**).
5. Wash bacteria by suspending pellet in an equal volume of DPBS and harvest by centrifugation at 3,000 × *g*, 4 °C for 10 min.
6. Resuspend bacteria in sterile DPBS to attain a final concentration of 2×10^8 colony-forming units (CFU)/mL.
7. Transfer bacterial suspension to septum vials and keep on ice until injection (*see* **Note 5**).
8. Verify the concentration of the bacterial inoculum by plating a 10^{-6} dilution on TSA plates.
9. Incubate the plates for 24 h at 37 °C and enumerate CFUs. This is a retrospective verification.

3.2 Preparation of Mice for Infection

Mice are shaved 1 day prior to inoculation to allow for enhanced visualization of the inoculation site and to obtain an accurate measurement of the abscess (*see* **Note 6**). All mouse procedures are performed under general anesthesia (*see* **Note 7**). The procedures described in this chapter conform to the guidelines set forth by the National Institutes of Health (NIH) and were reviewed and approved by the Institutional Animal Care and Use Committee (IACUC) at Rocky Mountain Laboratories, National Institute of Allergy and Infectious Diseases, NIH (*see* **Note 8**).

1. Anesthetize mice in an anesthesia chamber using the following settings: 2–2.5 % isoflurane and 2 L/min oxygen flow under standard atmospheric pressure (*see* **Note 9**).

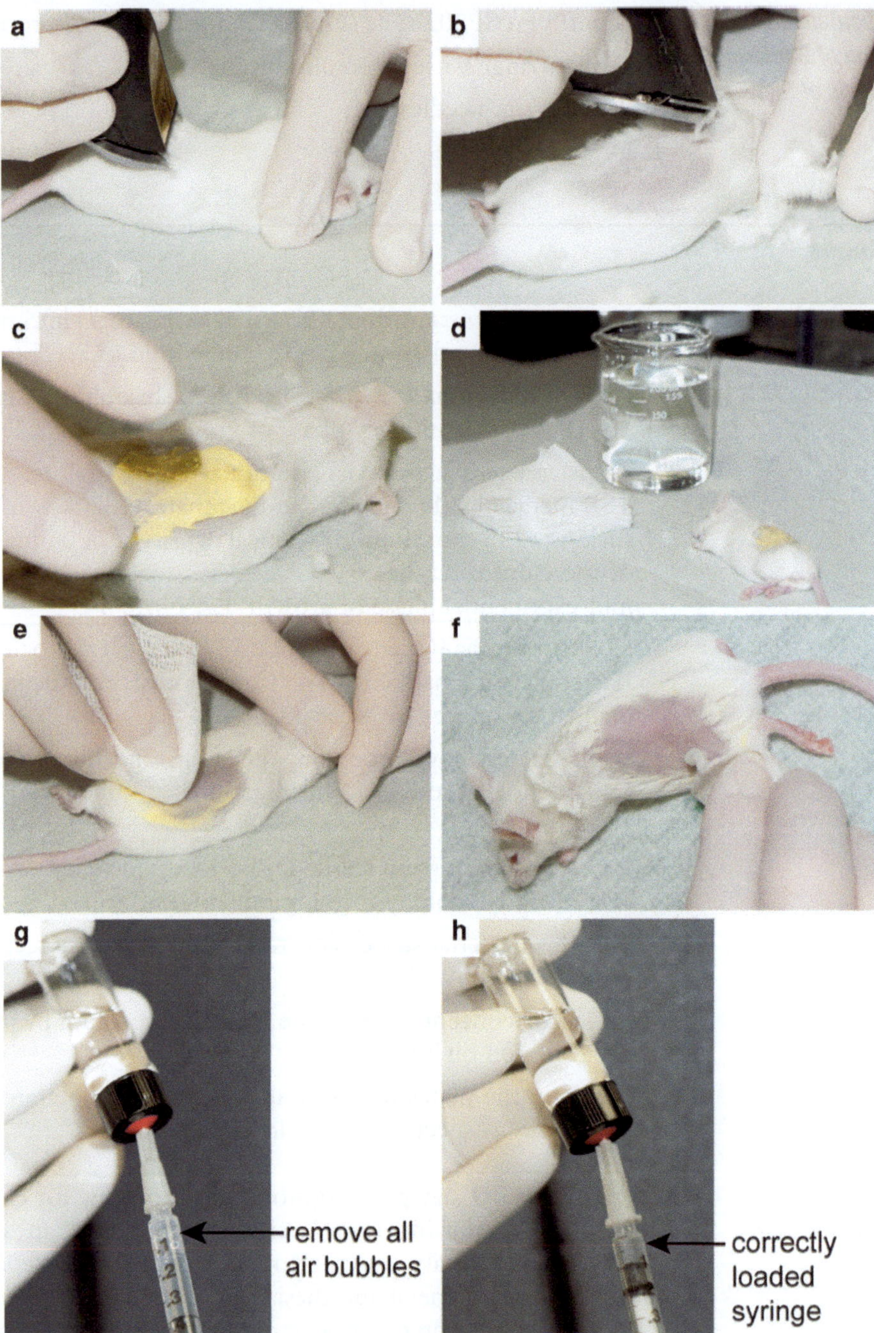

Fig. 1 Preparation of mice for infection. (**a** and **b**) Shaving a mouse with an electric trimmer. (**c**) Nair® is applied to remove remaining hairs and delay regrowth. (**d–f**) Removing Nair® with gauze pads and water. (**g** and **h**) Syringe loaded prior to expelling air bubbles (**g**) and after air bubbles were removed (**h**)

2. Remove animal from anesthesia chamber and carefully shave the infection site, typically the right and/or left flank, using an electric trimmer (Fig. 1a, b).

3. Cover the shaved area with Nair® for 3 min (see manufacturer instructions on the package for details) (*see* **Note 10**). Place the mouse into the anesthesia chamber during the 3-min incubation period (Fig. 1c).
4. Remove mouse from the anesthesia chamber and remove Nair® thoroughly using gauze sponges and water (Fig. 1d–f) (*see* **Note 11**).
5. At this point, animals should be marked with ear tattoos or ear punches to allow tracking and identification of individual animals.

3.3 Subcutaneous Inoculation

1. Anesthetize mice in an anesthesia chamber using the following settings: 2–2.5 % isoflurane and 2 L/min oxygen flow at under normal atmospheric pressure.
2. Weigh each mouse prior to inoculation (*see* **Note 12**).
3. Pinch the skin of the prepared site of infection to create a "tent" (Fig. 2a) (*see* **Note 13**).
4. Inoculate the animal subcutaneously with 0.05 mL of 1×10^7 live *S. aureus* or sterile saline (Fig. 2b) (*see* **Note 14**).

3.4 Monitoring the Course of Infection

1. The progression of disease, in this case abscess development, can be monitored by daily measurement of lesion dimensions and animal weight (*see* **Note 15**).
2. Measure the abscess length (L) and width (W) with the calipers (Fig. 2c, d). The abscess length and width dimensions are used to calculate the abscess volume [$V = 4/3\pi\ (L/2)^2 \times W/2$] and area [$A = \pi(L/2) \times W/2$] [19, 21].
3. Euthanize the animals at the end of the experiment (e.g., isoflurane overdose or CO_2 asphyxiation) (*see* **Note 16**).
4. Euthanized mice are bagged, labeled, and incinerated. Cages and bedding are autoclaved before washing.

4 Notes

1. The mouse SSTI infection model described in this chapter was developed for assessment of *S. aureus* virulence. However, this model can be adapted to test SSTI of other *S. aureus* strains and/or bacterial species.
2. Mouse strains are diverse and can vary by factors such as immunological features. Therefore, selection of the appropriate mouse strain should be considered carefully. For example, we frequently use Crl:SKH1-E hairless mice for the SSTI model, as animal preparation time is reduced (shaving and application of Nair are omitted) and skin lesions are easily measured.

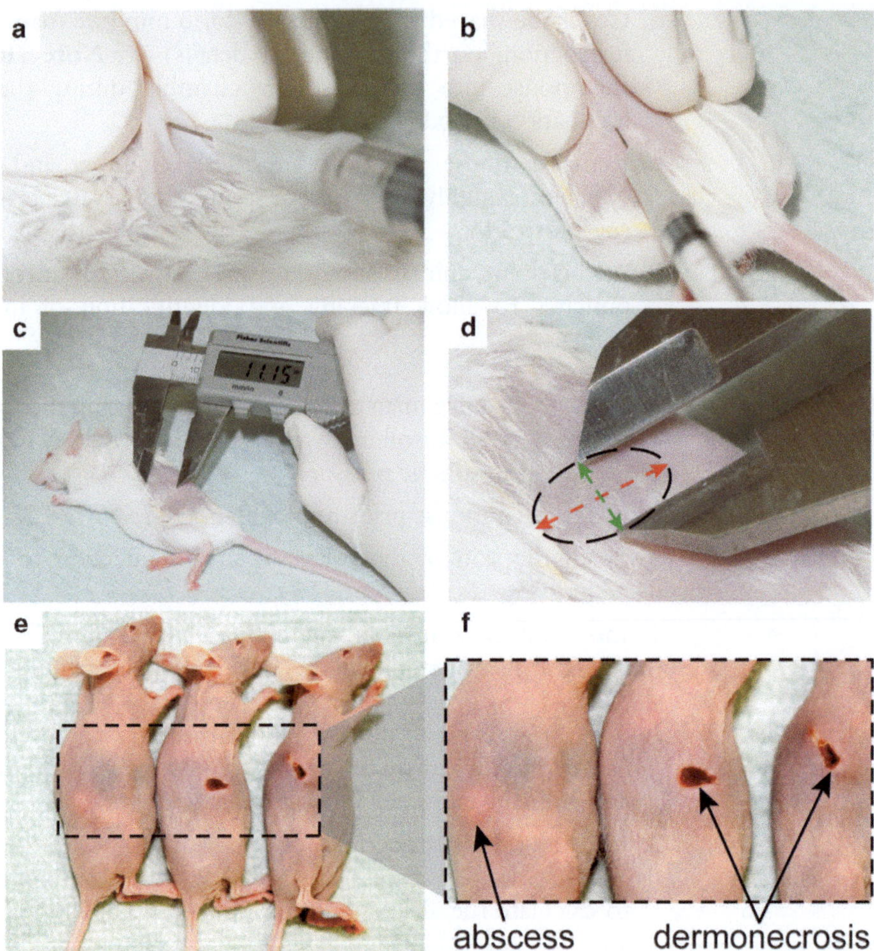

Fig. 2 Subcutaneous inoculation and subsequent analysis of skin lesions. (**a** and **b**) Subcutaneous injection. Panel (**a**) demonstrates formation of the "tent" when pinching the skin. (**c** and **d**) Taking measurements of the abscess area with calipers. (**d**) The "*green*" *arrow* represents the length that is measured in the "head-to-tail" direction of the animal and "*red*" is a width of the abscess or dermonecrosis area (dorsal–ventral). (**e**) Example of the abscess and dermonecrosis area on Day 4 post-injection (Crl:SKH1-E hairless mice). (**f**) A selected area from picture (**e**) is enlarged to improve visualization of lesion sites

3. The bacterial growth parameters used to generate the inoculum can be varied to suit the experimental hypothesis. In addition, frozen bacteria can be used to standardize the inoculum between different experiments. Changes in the inoculum may affect experimental outcome and should be vetted in pilot studies.
4. The total volume of bacteria for the injections should be calculated based on number of animals used per group. In our studies, we typically use 15 animals per test group and 5 animals for DPBS control based on guidance from statistical power analysis. See also **Note 5** for additional information.

5. For ease of loading syringes with the inoculum, we typically transfer three times the amount of bacterial inoculum that is required for all injections per test or control group to the septum vials. Excess inoculum is discarded following decontamination by autoclaving. Prolonged storage of the inoculum in DPBS on ice may reduce bacterial viability.
6. This step is unnecessary when using Crl:SKH1-E hairless mice.
7. All personnel entering the animal and procedure rooms must wear basic personal protective equipment, including laboratory coat, gloves, and facemask.
8. Animal care and use policies may vary by individual institution. Institutional policies and procedures regarding animal experimentation should be consulted prior to commencement of experimental design.
9. Isoflurane treatment may take up to 5 min to anesthetize mice sufficiently for the experimental procedures [22]. Depending on the experimental design, laboratory settings, or institutional requirements other inhalant or injectable anesthetics such as sevoflurane, ketamine or a combination of ketamine and xylazine may be substituted [23].
10. Nair® is applied to remove remaining hairs and prevent their regrowth for more accurate measurement of experimental lesions. Treatment should be performed at least 1 day prior to inoculation.
11. Either prolonged treatment or incomplete removal of Nair® will cause pronounced skin irritation and should be avoided.
12. A vessel to contain the mice is useful to facilitate manipulation of animals and to accurately assess weight.
13. The SSTI model can be modified to employ other modes of inoculation such as intradermal injection.
14. The optimal number of CFUs needed to achieve a reproducible SSTI should be determined in pilot experiments [18].
15. Typically, the subcutaneous injection of USA300 results in formation of a measurable abscess or area of dermonecrosis starting on days 2–3 with a maximum size achieved on ~day 6, followed by resolution of infection towards day 14 (Fig. 2e, f). Of note, the formation of dermonecrotic lesions is *S. aureus* strain and/or virulence factor specific [18, 20].
16. In our experience, local abscesses cause minimal pain or distress to the animals. However, should an abscess rupture, interfere with animal mobility, or mice show signs of disseminated disease (e.g., hunched posture, ruffled fur, reluctance to move, or not eating or drinking normally) they should be euthanized immediately.

Acknowledgments

The authors are supported by the Intramural Research Program of the National Institute of Allergy and Infectious Diseases, National Institutes of Health. The authors thank Anita Mora and Heather Murphy (Visual Information Specialist, RML/NIAID/NIH) for photography.

References

1. Kupper TS, Fuhlbrigge RC (2004) Immune surveillance in the skin: mechanisms and clinical consequences. Nat Rev Immunol 4:211–222
2. Nizet V, Ohtake T, Lauth X et al (2001) Innate antimicrobial peptide protects the skin from invasive bacterial infection. Nature 414:454–457
3. Lowell BA, Froelich CW, Federman DG et al (2001) Dermatology in primary care: prevalence and patient disposition. J Am Acad Dermatol 45:250–255
4. Sari F, Brian B, Brian M (2005) Skin disease in a primary care practice. Skinmed 4:350–353
5. Weinberg JM, Mysliwiec A, Turiansky GW et al (1997) Viral folliculitis: atypical presentations of herpes simplex, herpes zoster, and molluscum contagiosum. Arch Dermatol 133:983–986
6. Mika A, Goh P, Holt DC et al (2011) Scabies mite peritrophins are potential targets of human host innate immunity. PLoS Negl Trop Dis 5:e1331
7. Hengge UR, Currie BJ, Jäger G et al (2006) Scabies: a ubiquitous neglected skin disease. Lancet Infect Dis 6:769–779
8. Feldmeier H (2012) Pediculosis capitis: new insights into epidemiology, diagnosis and treatment. Eur J Clin Microbiol Infect Dis. doi:10.1007/s10096-012-1575-0
9. Saracino A, Kelly R, Liew D et al (2011) Pyoderma gangrenosum requiring inpatient management: a report of 26 cases with follow up. Australas J Dermatol 52:218–221
10. Shim TN, Lew TT, Preston PW (2012) Disseminated cutaneous Mycobacterium chelonae. Lancet Infect Dis 12:254
11. Pallin DJ, Espinola JA, Leung DY et al (2009) Epidemiology of dermatitis and skin infections in United States physicians' offices, 1993–2005. Clin Infect Dis 49:901–907
12. Talan DA, Krishnadasan A, Gorwitz RJ et al (2011) Comparison of Staphylococcus aureus from skin and soft-tissue infections in US emergency department patients, 2004 and 2008. Clin Infect Dis 53:144–149
13. Fridkin SK, Hageman JC, Morrison M et al (2005) Methicillin-resistant Staphylococcus aureus disease in three communities. N Engl J Med 352:1436–1444
14. Moran GJ, Krishnadasan A, Gorwitz RJ et al (2006) Methicillin-resistant S. aureus infections among patients in the emergency department. N Engl J Med 355:666–674
15. Watts A, Ke D, Wang Q et al (2005) Staphylococcus aureus strains that express serotype 5 or serotype 8 capsular polysaccharides differ in virulence. Infect Immun 73:3502–3511
16. Hoebe K, Georgel P, Rutschmann S et al (2005) CD36 is a sensor of diacylglycerides. Nature 433:523–527
17. Hume EB, Cole N, Khan S et al (2005) A Staphylococcus aureus mouse keratitis topical infection model: cytokine balance in different strains of mice. Immunol Cell Biol 83:294–300
18. Voyich JM, Otto M, Mathema B et al (2006) Is Panton-Valentine leukocidin the major virulence determinant in community-associated methicillin-resistant Staphylococcus aureus disease? J Infect Dis 194:1761–1770
19. Bunce C, Wheeler L, Reed G et al (1992) Murine model of cutaneous infection with gram-positive cocci. Infect Immun 60: 2636–2640
20. Kennedy AD, Wardenburg JB, Gardner DJ et al (2010) Targeting of alpha-hemolysin by active or passive immunization decreases severity of USA300 skin infection in a mouse model. J Infect Dis 202:1050–1058
21. Lukomski S, Montgomery CA, Rurangirwa J et al (1999) Extracellular cysteine protease produced by Streptococcus pyogenes participates in the pathogenesis of invasive skin infection and dissemination in mice. Infect Immun 67:1779–1788
22. Cesarovic N, Nicholls F, Rettich A et al (2010) Isoflurane and sevoflurane provide equally effective anaesthesia in laboratory mice. Lab Anim 44:329–336
23. Gaertner DJ, Hallman TM, Hankenson FC et al (2008) Anesthesia and analgesia for laboratory rodents. In: Richard EF, Marilyn JB, Peggy JD et al (eds) Anesthesia and analgesia in laboratory animals, 2nd edn. Academic Press, San Diego, pp 239–297

Chapter 15

Sepsis Induced by Cecal Ligation and Puncture

Haitao Wen

Abstract

Despite advances in intensive care unit interventions, including the use of specific antibiotics and anti-inflammation treatment, sepsis with concomitant multiple organ failure is the most common cause of death in many acute care units. In order to understand the mechanisms of clinical sepsis and develop effective therapeutic modalities, there is a need to use effective experimental models that faithfully replicate what occurs in patients with sepsis. Several models are commonly used to study sepsis, including intravenous endotoxin challenge, injection of live organisms into the peritoneal cavity, establishing abscesses in the extremities, and the induction of polymicrobial peritonitis via cecal ligation and puncture (CLP). Here, we describe the surgery procedure of CLP in mice, which has been proposed to closely replicate the nature and course of clinical sepsis in humans.

Key words Sepsis, Cecal ligation and puncture, CLP, Cytokine, Macrophage

1 Introduction

Sepsis, caused by gram-negative (G^-) and gram-positive (G^+) bacteria, fungi, viruses, and parasites, has become increasingly significant over the past decades. This condition affects approximately 700,000 people annually and accounts for about 210,000 deaths per year in the USA [1–5]. Despite technical developments in intensive care units (ICUs) and advanced supportive treatment, the incidence of sepsis is rising at rates between 1.5 and 8 % per year [4, 5]. These rates may be caused by the increased usage of catheters and other invasive instruments, chemotherapy for cancer patients, and immunosuppression in patients with organ transplants or inflammatory diseases. Sepsis represents a major burden to the US health care system, with costs of approximately $16.7 billion per year, due in part to the extended hospitalization of septic patients [4]. Interestingly, the contribution of G^+ bacteria to sepsis has dramatically increased during the past 30 years [5], with *Staphylococcus aureus* and *S. epidermidis* being responsible for more than half of these cases of sepsis [6, 7]. In addition, the rate of

Irving C. Allen (ed.), *Mouse Models of Innate Immunity: Methods and Protocols*, Methods in Molecular Biology, vol. 1031, DOI 10.1007/978-1-62703-481-4_15, © Springer Science+Business Media, LLC 2013

Table 1
Sepsis diagnostic criteria

General changes	Hyperthermia (>38.3 °C) or hypothermia (<36 °C) Heart rate >90/min or >2 SD above normal value for age Breath rate >30/min Changes in mental state Edema or positive fluid balance (>20 ml/kg over 24 h) Plasma glucose >120 mg/dl or >7.7 mM
Inflammatory changes	WBC $>12\times10^9$/l or $< 4\times10^9$/l Normal WBC count with >10 % immature band forms Plasma C reactive protein >2 SD above normal Plasma procalcitonin >2 SD above normal
Hemodynamic changes	Arterial hypotension (SBP <90 mmHg, MAP <70, or a SBP decrease >40 in adults or <2 SD below the normal for age) SvO_2 >70 % Cardiac index >3.5 L/min/M^{-23}
Organ dysfunction	Arterial hypoxemia (PaO_2/FiO_2 <300) Acute oliguria (urine output <0.5 ml/kg/h or <45 mM for at least 2 h) Creatinine increase >0.5 mg/dl Coagulation abnormalities (INR >1.5 or aPPT >60 s) Ileus (absent bowel sounds) Platelet count <100,000/μl Plasma total bilirubin >4 mg/dl or >70 mM
Tissue perfusion	Serum lactate level >1 mM Decreased capillary refill

WBC white blood cell, *SBP* systolic blood pressure, *MAP* mean arterial pressure, *SvO_2* mixed venous oxygen saturation, *PaO_2* arterial partial pressure of oxygen, *FiO_2* fraction of inspired oxygen, *INR* international normalized ratio, *aPPT* activated partial thromboplastin time

fungal infections is reported to have increased more than 200 % [5]. The clinical definition of sepsis has been continuously modified based on additional clinical symptoms and laboratory findings. Discussion at the most recent consensus conference led to the establishment of the extended definition of sepsis, which is outlined in Table 1 [8–10].

During the initiation and progression of sepsis, two dynamic stages are present; a systemic inflammatory response syndrome (SIRS) in the acute phase and a compensatory anti-inflammatory response syndrome (CARS) in the later phase [9]. The hallmark of SIRS/CARS is an exacerbated production of pro-and anti-inflammatory cytokines/chemokines, leading to the so-called cytokine storm. While these inflammatory mediators are essential in providing an effective host defense, their overzealous production can be deleterious, resulting in a "double-edge sword" property of reducing pathogens at the expense of organ injury [11, 12]. In the host, toll-like receptors (TLRs) and intracellular pattern recognition receptors (PRRs), such as nucleotide-binding oligomerization domain (NOD)-leuine-rich repeat (LRR) family (NOD-LRR) proteins, act as sensors for invading pathogens or their components. Activation of these sensors results in the release of an array of proinflammatory mediators from both leukocytes and structural cells. These mediators include, but are not limited to, tumor necrosis factor (TNF)-α, interleukin (IL)-1β, IL-6, CXCL8 (IL-8), IL-18, CCL2 (MCP-1), CCL3 (MIP-1α), CXCL10 (IP-10) [10, 11, 13, 14], prostaglandins, lipid mediators, and reactive oxygen species [7]. The effects of these host-derived factors include vasodilatation and upregulation of adhesion molecules, resulting in the extravasation of leukocytes and the activation of these cells along with epithelial and endothelial cells. Coagulation is an additional vascular event that is dictated directly by pathogen components and indirectly by pathogen-induced cytokines. This physiological response can be more severe and result in disseminated intravascular coagulation (DIC), causing hypoperfusion, hypoxia and death. Collectively, the tissue damage caused by activated immune cells and pathological coagulation resulting in DIC can lead to multiple organ failure (MOF), involving the lungs (acute respiratory distress syndrome), liver, and kidneys [2, 15–17]. Based on the understanding of molecular mechanisms underlying sepsis, new clinical therapies have been designed to neutralize several key molecules involved in the initiation and progression of sepsis, including lipopolysaccharide (LPS), a core component of G^- bacteria cell wall, IL-1, and TNF-α. Although experimental studies using animal models of sepsis have documented a beneficial effect of these therapies [18–22], subsequent clinical trials were disappointing since they showed no substantial benefits [23–27]. So far, recombinant human activated protein C that targets coagulation remains the only effective new therapy for clinically severe sepsis [28]. These observations support the concept that severe sepsis is a highly dynamic and complex disorder and efficient treatment strategies remain elusive.

In order to understand the mechanisms of clinical sepsis and develop effective therapeutic modalities, there is a need to use effective experimental models that faithfully replicate what occurs in patients with sepsis. Several models, including endotoxin challenge, live organism challenge, establishing abscesses in the extremities, and the induction of polymicrobial peritonitis via cecal ligation and puncture (CLP) have been used to study sepsis [29–31]. The latter experimental model, CLP, has been proposed to more closely replicate the nature and course of clinical sepsis, as compared to other models [32, 33]. The benefits of the CLP model is its reproducibility and the potential to alter the severity of sepsis by controlling needle size, number of cecal punctures and antibiotic utilization [34]. Following the induction of CLP-induced peritonitis, inflammatory cytokines/chemokines such as IL-12p70, IL-10, TNF-α, CCL2, CCL3, and CXCL10 are rapidly induced in the peritoneal cavity (local response), blood and peripheral organs (systemic response) within 4 h and peak at 24 h. Three days later, the local and systemic levels of inflammatory cytokines/chemokines mostly return to baseline levels, indicating the end of the acute phase of sepsis.

2 Materials

2.1 Animals

1. Female C57BL/6 mice (6–8 weeks; The Jackson Laboratory) housed under specific pathogen-free conditions (*see* **Note 1**).

2.2 Surgical Supplies and Equipment

1. 3-0 silk suture.
2. Autoclip wound closing system, including applier.
3. Wound clips and remover.
4. Scissors and forceps.
5. Heating pad.
6. 5 ml syringe.
7. 21-gauge needles.
8. Instant sealing sterilization pouch.

2.3 Reagents

1. Ketamine HCl (Abbott Laboratories).
2. Xylazine (Lloyd Laboratories).
3. Antibiotic INVANZ (Ertapenem) (Merck).
4. Sterile saline (Hospira).
5. Veterinary ointment (Pharmaderm).

3 Methods (*see* Note 2)

1. Autoclave all of the surgical equipment, including the scissors, forceps, and wound clips, with the Instant Sealing Sterilization Pouch.
2. Prior to CLP surgery, anesthetize the mice with a combination of 2.25 mg of ketamine and 150 μg of xylazine administrated intraperitoneally. Once the mice are anesthetized, apply moisturizing vet ointment to the eyes to prevent drying.
3. Under sterile surgical conditions, a 1-cm midline incision is made to the ventral surface of the abdomen, and the cecum is exposed (Fig. 1a).

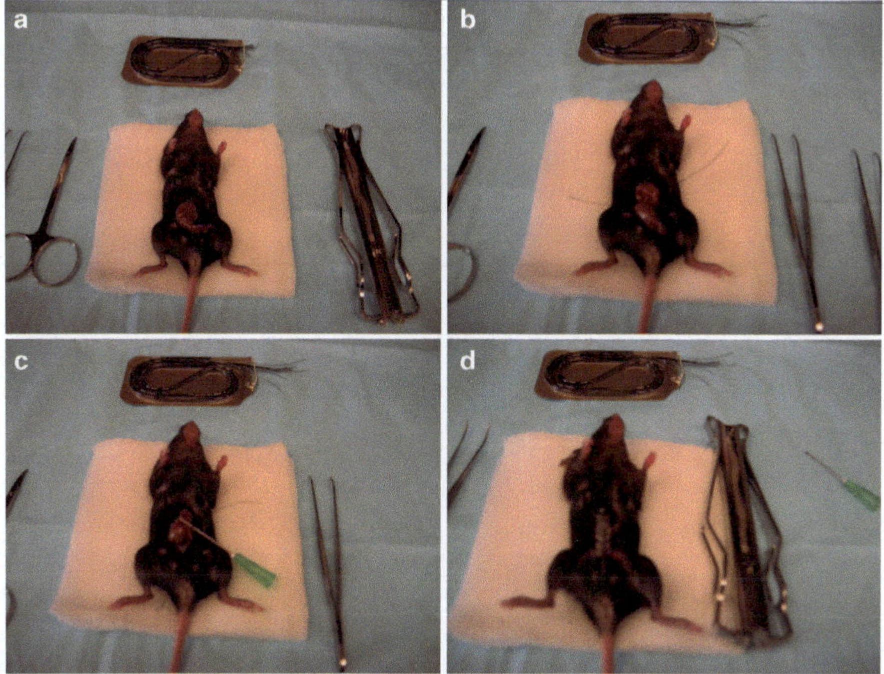

Fig. 1 Cecal ligation and puncture procedure (**a**) A 1-cm midline incision is made by scissor to the ventral surface of the abdomen, and the cecum is exposed. (**b**) The cecum is partially ligated at its base with a 3-0 silk suture. (**c**) The ligated cecum is punctured up to nine times with 21-gauge needle. (**d**) The cecum is returned to the peritoneal cavity and the abdominal incision was closed using two or three surgical wound clips

4. The cecum is partially ligated at its base with a 3-0 silk suture (Fig. 1b).
5. The ligated cecum is punctured up to nine times with a 21-gauge needle (Fig. 1c). Sham-operated mice will undergo an identical operation except for the actual CLP. These sham-operated mice will serve as controls.
6. The cecum is returned to the peritoneal cavity and the abdominal incision is closed using two or three surgical wound clips (Fig. 1d).
7. Immediately administer 1 ml of sterile saline subcutaneously to each mouse for fluid resuscitation.
8. Allow the mice to recover from anesthesia in a face-down position in a bedding-free, pre-warmed fresh cage placed over a heating pad. Monitor the cage temperature to prevent overheating. It usually takes about 30 min for mice to recover from anesthesia.
9. Treat both CLP and sham mice with the antibiotic INVANZ (Ertapenem). INVANZ should be administered intraperitoneally at 75 mg/kg beginning at 6 h after surgery and reinjected every 24 h until day 3 post-surgery.

10. Disease progression should be monitored three times per day by evaluating weight loss, temperature decrease, and behavioral changes. Monitor the animal survival for 6 days.
11. Peritoneal lavage, serum, and various tissues such as lung, liver, and kidney are collected at day 1 or day 3 for cytokine measurement.

4 Notes

1. The genetic background of the animals is important. In contrast to T helper (Th) 2-dominant BALB/c mice, C57BL/6 mice are Th1-dominant and more resistant to trauma-induced sepsis [35] and Th1-dependent pathological infections, such as *Leishmania major* [36, 37]. Thus, female C57BL/6 mice were used extensively as an animal of choice for inducing experimental sepsis. On average, this nine-puncture CLP procedure results in approximately 40 % mortality in the acute phase of sepsis [38–40].
2. All studies must be conducted in accordance with the local and institutional animal care and use guidelines and in accord with the prevailing national regulations.

Acknowledgments

Haitao Wen is supported by the Postdoctoral Fellowship of the American Heart Association, Mid-Atlantic Affiliate and Postdoctoral Fellowship of the Cancer Research Institute.

References

1. Glauser MP, Zanetti G, Baumgartner JD, Cohen J (1991) Septic shock: pathogenesis. Lancet 338:732–736
2. Parrillo JE (1993) Pathogenetic mechanisms of septic shock. N Engl J Med 328: 1471–1477
3. Opal SM, Cohen J (1999) Clinical gram-positive sepsis: does it fundamentally differ from gram-negative bacterial sepsis? Crit Care Med 27:1608–1616
4. Angus DC, Linde-Zwirble WT, Lidicker J, Clermont G, Carcillo J, Pinsky MR (2001) Epidemiology of severe sepsis in the United States: analysis of incidence, outcome, and associated costs of care. Crit Care Med 29:1303–1310
5. Martin GS, Mannino DM, Eaton S, Moss M (2003) The epidemiology of sepsis in the United States from 1979 through 2000. N Engl J Med 348:1546–1554
6. Geerdes HF, Ziegler D, Lode H, Hund M, Loehr A, Fangmann W, Wagner J (1992) Septicemia in 980 patients at a university hospital in Berlin: prospective studies during 4 selected years between 1979 and 1989. Clin Infect Dis 15:991–1002
7. Van Amersfoort ES, Van Berkel TJ, Kuiper J (2003) Receptors, mediators, and mechanisms involved in bacterial sepsis and septic shock. Clin Microbiol Rev 16:379–414
8. Levy MM, Fink MP, Marshall JC, Abraham E, Angus D, Cook D, Cohen J, Opal SM, Vincent

JL, Ramsay G (2003) 2001 SCCM/ESICM/ACCP/ATS/SIS international sepsis definitions conference. Intensive Care Med 29: 530–538

9. Riedemann NC, Guo RF, Ward PA (2003) The enigma of sepsis. J Clin Invest 112: 460–467
10. Tschoeke SK, Oberholzer A, Moldawer LL (2006) Interleukin-18: a novel prognostic cytokine in bacteria-induced sepsis. Crit Care Med 34:1225–1233
11. Cavaillon JM, Adib-Conquy M, Fitting C, Adrie C, Payen D (2003) Cytokine cascade in sepsis. Scand J Infect Dis 35:535–544
12. Lin WJ, Yeh WC (2005) Implication of toll-like receptor and tumor necrosis factor alpha signaling in septic shock. Shock 24:206–209
13. Lin KJ, Lin J, Hanasawa K, Tani T, Kodama M (2000) Interleukin-8 as a predictor of the severity of bacteremia and infectious disease. Shock 14:95–100
14. Coelho AL, Hogaboam CM, Kunkel SL (2005) Chemokines provide the sustained inflammatory bridge between innate and acquired immunity. Cytokine Growth Factor Rev 16:553–560
15. Horn KD (1998) Evolving strategies in the treatment of sepsis and systemic inflammatory response syndrome (SIRS). Qjm 91:265–277
16. Karima R, Matsumoto S, Higashi H, Matsushima K (1999) The molecular pathogenesis of endotoxic shock and organ failure. Mol Med Today 5:123–132
17. Riedemann NC, Guo RF, Ward PA (2003) Novel strategies for the treatment of sepsis. Nat Med 9:517–524
18. Davis CE, Brown KR, Douglas H, Tate WJ 3rd, Braude AI (1969) Prevention of death from endotoxin with antisera. I. The risk of fatal anaphylaxis to endotoxin. J Immunol 102:563–572
19. Beutler B, Milsark IW, Cerami AC (1985) Passive immunization against cachectin/tumor necrosis factor protects mice from lethal effect of endotoxin. Science 229:869–871
20. Tracey KJ, Beutler B, Lowry SF, Merryweather J, Wolpe S, Milsark IW, Hariri RJ, Fahey TJ 3rd, Zentella A, Albert JD et al (1986) Shock and tissue injury induced by recombinant human cachectin. Science 234:470–474
21. Tracey KJ, Fong Y, Hesse DG, Manogue KR, Lee AT, Kuo GC, Lowry SF, Cerami A (1987) Anti-cachectin/TNF monoclonal antibodies prevent septic shock during lethal bacteraemia. Nature 330:662–664
22. Ohlsson K, Bjork P, Bergenfeldt M, Hageman R, Thompson RC (1990) Interleukin-1 receptor antagonist reduces mortality from endotoxin shock. Nature 348:550–552
23. Cohen J (1999) Adjunctive therapy in sepsis: a critical analysis of the clinical trial programme. Br Med Bull 55:212–225
24. Reinhart K, Karzai W (2001) Anti-tumor necrosis factor therapy in sepsis: update on clinical trials and lessons learned. Crit Care Med 29:S121–S125
25. Fisher CJ Jr, Agosti JM, Opal SM, Lowry SF, Balk RA, Sadoff JC, Abraham E, Schein RM, Benjamin E (1996) Treatment of septic shock with the tumor necrosis factor receptor:Fc fusion protein. The Soluble TNF Receptor Sepsis Study Group. N Engl J Med 334: 1697–1702
26. Fisher CJ Jr, Dhainaut JF, Opal SM, Pribble JP, Balk RA, Slotman GJ, Iberti TJ, Rackow EC, Shapiro MJ, Greenman RL et al (1994) Recombinant human interleukin 1 receptor antagonist in the treatment of patients with sepsis syndrome. Results from a randomized, double-blind, placebo-controlled trial. Phase III rhIL-1ra Sepsis Syndrome Study Group. JAMA 271:1836–1843
27. Opal SM, Fisher CJ Jr, Dhainaut JF, Vincent JL, Brase R, Lowry SF, Sadoff JC, Slotman GJ, Levy H, Balk RA et al (1997) Confirmatory interleukin-1 receptor antagonist trial in severe sepsis: a phase III, randomized, double-blind, placebo-controlled, multicenter trial. The Interleukin-1 Receptor Antagonist Sepsis Investigator Group. Crit Care Med 25: 1115–1124
28. Bernard GR, Vincent JL, Laterre PF, LaRosa SP, Dhainaut JF, Lopez-Rodriguez A, Steingrub JS, Garber GE, Helterbrand JD, Ely EW et al (2001) Efficacy and safety of recombinant human activated protein C for severe sepsis. N Engl J Med 344:699–709
29. Deitch EA (1998) Animal models of sepsis and shock: a review and lessons learned. Shock 9:1–11
30. Parker SJ, Watkins PE (2001) Experimental models of gram-negative sepsis. Br J Surg 88:22–30
31. Esmon CT (2004) Why do animal models (sometimes) fail to mimic human sepsis? Crit Care Med 32:S219–222
32. Maier S, Traeger T, Entleutner M, Westerholt A, Kleist B, Huser N, Holzmann B, Stier A, Pfeffer K, Heidecke CD (2004) Cecal ligation and puncture versus colon ascendens stent peritonitis: two distinct animal models for polymicrobial sepsis. Shock 21:505–511
33. Hubbard WJ, Choudhry M, Schwacha MG, Kerby JD, Rue LW 3rd, Bland KI, Chaudry IH (2005) Cecal ligation and puncture. Shock 24(Suppl 1):52–57
34. Walley KR, Lukacs NW, Standiford TJ, Strieter RM, Kunkel SL (1996) Balance of inflammatory

cytokines related to severity and mortality of murine sepsis. Infect Immun 64:4733–4738
35. Radojicic C, Andric B, Simovic M, Dujic A, Marinkovic D (1990) Genetic basis of resistance to trauma in inbred strains of mice. J Trauma 30:211–213
36. von Stebut E, Udey MC (2004) Requirements for Th1-dependent immunity against infection with Leishmania major. Microbes Infect 6:1102–1109
37. Sacks D, Noben-Trauth N (2002) The immunology of susceptibility and resistance to Leishmania major in mice. Nat Rev Immunol 2:845–858
38. Benjamim CF, Hogaboam CM, Lukacs NW, Kunkel SL (2003) Septic mice are susceptible to pulmonary aspergillosis. Am J Pathol 163:2605–2617
39. Benjamim CF, Lundy SK, Lukacs NW, Hogaboam CM, Kunkel SL (2005) Reversal of long-term sepsis-induced immunosuppression by dendritic cells. Blood 105: 3588–3595
40. Wen H, Hogaboam CM, Gauldie J, Kunkel SL (2006) Severe sepsis exacerbates cell-mediated immunity in the lung due to an altered dendritic cell cytokine profile. Am J Pathol 168:1940–1950

Chapter 16

Systemic Infection of Mice with *Listeria monocytogenes* to Characterize Host Immune Responses

Nancy Wang, Richard A. Strugnell, Odilia L. Wijburg, and Thomas C. Brodnicki

Abstract

Listeria monocytogenes is a Gram-positive facultative intracellular bacterium that is widely used to characterize bacterial pathogenesis and host immunity. Here, we describe a set of basic methods and techniques to infect mice with *L. monocytogenes*, measure bacterial load in tissues, and analyze immune cell subsets responding to infection in the spleen and liver. In addition, a specialized method for immune cell depletion is incorporated within the overall protocol, along with suggestions at various points in the protocol for minimizing experimental variability in mouse infection studies using *L. monocytogenes*. Finally, we highlight a number of experimental strategies for which *L. monocytogenes* has facilitated research into host immune responses and bacterial pathogenesis.

Key words *Listeria*, Intracellular bacterium, Mouse, Liver, Spleen, Blood, Lymphocytes, Neutrophils, Host immune response, Genetic susceptibility, Flow cytometry, Fluorescence-activated cell sorting

1 Introduction

Listeria monocytogenes is a widely used intracellular pathogen for investigating genetic factors, immune cell subsets, and molecular mechanisms that are important for host immune responses to bacterial infection [1–4]. Systemic infection using *L. monocytogenes* in mouse models is typically achieved by intravenous injection, which leads to rapid dissemination and subsequent proliferation of the bacteria in the spleen and liver [5, 6]. Intravenous injection also elicits highly synchronized and coordinated responses from innate and adaptive immune cells [1, 4, 7]. Various innate immune cells (e.g., dendritic cells, Kuppfer cells, monocytes, neutrophils, NK cells) respond within the first few days of infection to control bacterial proliferation. Activation of the innate immune system facilitates the development of an adaptive immune response, predominantly mediated by $CD8^+$ T cells, that leads to the eventual clearance of

Irving C. Allen (ed.), *Mouse Models of Innate Immunity: Methods and Protocols*, Methods in Molecular Biology, vol. 1031, DOI 10.1007/978-1-62703-481-4_16, © Springer Science+Business Media, LLC 2013

L. monocytogenes from the host, typically within 10 days of infection. Advantages of working with this bacterium include: it is easy to culture in the lab; the genomic sequences of *L. monocytogenes* and related species are known [8]; a number of mutant strains that differentially probe host immune responses have been described [9, 10]; and *L. monocytogenes*-derived epitopes, recognized by $CD4^+$ and, more importantly, $CD8^+$ T cells, have been defined and demonstrate strong immunodominance in certain inbred mouse strains [11]. Additional reviews describe these and other features of *L. monocytogenes* that facilitate research using this bacterium [12–16].

This protocol consists of four general methods: (1) preparation and storage of infectious *L. monocytogenes* stocks, (2) infection of mice, (3) measurement of bacterial load in tissues, and (4) generation of splenic and hepatic single-cell suspensions for FACS analysis of immune cell subsets. A specialized method for in vivo depletion of specific immune cell subsets is also incorporated within this protocol to identify the roles of cells expressing specific surface markers during *L. monocytogenes* infection. In addition, a number of precautions are described in the accompanying notes to minimize unwanted variability when measuring bacterial load and immune responses. For example, *L. monocytogenes* should be obtained from a proven source and inocula prepared from fresh overnight cultures to optimize viability and relative virulence between experiments. To control for variability within an experiment, the concentration of the inoculum (colony forming units [CFU]/ml) should be determined before and after injecting mice to confirm that the number of bacteria does not differ greatly between the first and last mouse injected. Another important step is perfusion of the liver, which depletes circulating leukocytes and ensures accurate measurement of immune cells within the liver. If a cell-depleting antibody is to be used, it is necessary to determine the effective dose that will deplete the chosen immune cell type for the desired time period. These steps, along with other suggestions and precautions, for a typical mouse infection study are more fully covered in the detailed protocol and 4 Notes below.

L. monocytogenes infection in mice provides a number of experimental strategies for investigating the molecular and cellular components of the immune system [1, 2]. In the first instance, *L. monocytogenes* infection provides a relatively straightforward test of how well the immune system for a chosen mouse strain (e.g., knockout mouse) responds to an intracellular infection. Bacterial load and clearance can be measured in the liver and spleen post-infection by culturing tissue homogenate on blood agar plates and counting the number of CFU. Generally, susceptible inbred mouse strains with genetically deficient immune responses to *L. monocytogenes* will have higher bacterial loads and/or delayed bacterial clearance compared with resistant mouse strains. The protocol presented here also enables the measurement of bacterial load and immune cell responses within a single tissue of a given mouse. This dual measurement of a particular tissue for each infected mouse provides for more robust comparisons within and between mouse cohorts (either representing different mouse strains or time points post-infection). The resulting single-cell suspensions can also be used for a variety of analyses, including measuring and isolating immune cell subsets, and in vitro characterization of sorted immune cells from infected mice [17, 18]. More complex studies, such as cell depletion or linkage analyses of mouse intercrosses, can be employed to identify the effects of particular immune cells or sequence variation for genes that affect host immune responses to *L. monocytogenes* infection [19–25]. Alternatively, this protocol can be readily adapted to compare infection of mice with different *L. monocytogenes* strains to identify bacterial virulence factors that are important for specific host–pathogen interactions [26, 27]. It can also be adapted to characterize the potential of recombinant *L. monocytogenes* to serve as a live vector for vaccine delivery [28, 29]. In summary, this protocol provides the basic methods and techniques required to perform experiments investigating *L. monocytogenes* pathogenesis and host immune responses in mice.

2 Materials

Prepare all solutions using ultrapure water (prepared by purifying deionized water to attain a sensitivity of 18 MΩ at 22 °C) and analytical grade reagents. Prepare and store all reagents at room temperature, unless otherwise indicated.

2.1 *Listeria monocytogenes*

1. Culture *Listeria monocytogenes*. When cultured on blood agar, *L. monocytogenes* exhibits a characteristic halo zone around each colony due to β-hemolysis caused by *Listeria*-secreted protein listeriolysin O (Fig. 1a [30]). Different *L. monocytogenes* strains may vary significantly for virulence and result in different infection kinetics and/or immune responses in infected mice. It is recommended that each new strain of *L. monocytogenes* be tested for determination of the optimal sublethal dose for a particular mouse strain (*see* **Note 1**). Some of the most commonly used virulent strains include EGD, 10403s (resistant to streptomycin) and 43251. The methods described here can be used with virulent and avirulent *L. monocytogenes* strains. While good bacteriological practice should ensure "clonality" of cultures, contaminating growth in the culture can be eliminated by supplementing growth media with antibiotics (to which the *Listeria sp.* are resistant) or through the use of Oxford media formulation for selective culture of *L. monocytogenes* strains (Fig. 1b [32]).

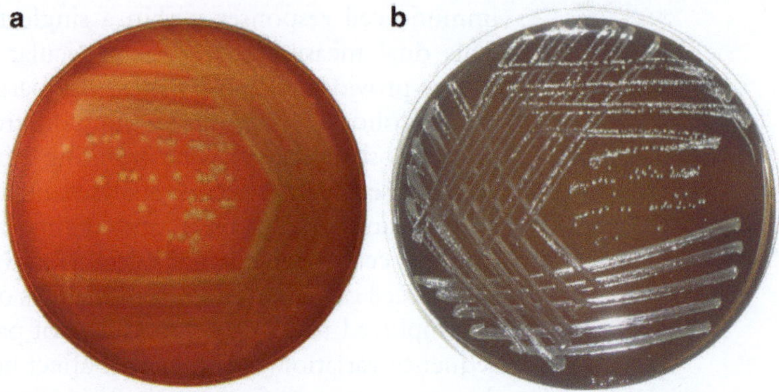

Fig. 1 *L. monocytogenes* streaked onto HBA plates. Using a sterile inoculating loop, *L. monocytogenes* was streaked over ¼ of the plate surface as the primary inoculum spread, followed by 2–3 unidirectional streaks from the primary spread. A fresh or re-sterilized loop was used before each set of streaks so that individual colonies could be observed after incubating the plates at 37 °C overnight. (**a**) After 24-h growth at 37 °C, a characteristic halo zone around each *L. monocytogenes* colony is observed on the HBA plates, as viewed from the bottom of the agar plate with back lighting. (**b**) Typical appearance of *L. monocytogenes* colonies after 40-h of growth at 37 °C on Oxford agar plates, as viewed from the top of the plate

2.2 Media for Growing *L. monocytogenes*

1. Horse blood agar (HBA) plates: Use Oxoid CM0271 (agar base) and HB1000 (horse blood); or alternatively use 15 g of proteose peptone, 2.5 g of liver digest, 5 g of yeast extract, 5 g of sodium chloride, and 12 g of agar to make 1 L of agar base in water, pH 7.2 ± 0.2 at 25 °C; supplement with 7 % sterile horse blood.
2. Brain heart infusion (BHI) broth: Use Oxoid CM1135; or alternatively use 12.5 g of brain infusion solids, 5 g of beef heart infusion solids, 10 g of proteose peptone, 2 g of glucose, 5 g of sodium chloride, and 2.5 g of disodium phosphate to make 1 L in water, pH 7.4 ± 0.2 at 25 °C.
3. Oxford agar plates (optional): Use Oxoid CM0856 (agar base) and SR0140 (supplement); or alternatively use 23 g of peptone, 1 g of starch, 5 g of sodium chloride, 10 g of agar, 1 g of aesculin, 0.5 g of ferric ammonium citrate, and 15 g of lithium chloride to make 1 L of agar base in water, pH 7.0 ± 0.2 at 25 °C; supplement per liter with 400 mg of cycloheximide, 20 mg of colistsin sulfate, 5 mg of acriflavine, 2 mg of cefotetan, and 10 mg of fosfomycin.

2.3 Solutions

1. 80 % (v/v) glycerol.
2. 80 % (v/v) ethanol.
3. PBS: 0.24 g of potassium chloride, 0.2 g of potassium dihydrogen phosphate, 8 g of sodium chloride, 1.44 g of disodium hydrogen phosphate, prepared in 1 L of water, pH 7.2–7.4.

4. FACS buffer: 0.1 % (w/v) bovine serum albumin in PBS.
5. Isotonic Percoll: 67.5 mL of Percoll, 7.5 mL of 10× PBS, 125 mL of 1× PBS, makes 200 mL.
6. TAC buffer: 17 mM Tris, 140 mM ammonium chloride in water, pH 7.2.
7. FCS/EDTA buffer: Fetal calf serum with 10 mM EDTA.
8. FACS/EDTA buffer: FACS buffer with 5 mM EDTA.
9. Trypan blue cell staining solution: 0.4 % (w/v) trypan blue powder in ultrapure water.

2.4 Consumables

1. Inoculating loop.
2. 30 mL McCartney bottle.
3. Glass or plastic spreader for spreading bacteria on agar plates.
4. Cuvettes for the spectrophotometer.
5. 1.5 mL microfuge tubes.
6. Cryovials.
7. Syringes: 1, 5, and 10 mL.
8. Needles: 25, 26, and 27 gauge.
9. 60 mm and 90 mm petri dish.
10. 50 mL conical screw-cap tube.
11. 10 mL centrifuge tube.
12. 70 μm cell strainer.
13. 100 μm nylon membrane.
14. Stomacher bag.
15. 96-well flat bottom plate.
16. Lithium heparin-coated Vacutainer tubes.

2.5 Equipment

1. Orbital shaker incubator for liquid bacterial cultures.
2. Spectrophotometer.
3. 150 W infrared lamp.
4. Hemocytometer.
5. Microscope.
6. Stomacher (Seward, UK).

3 Methods (*See* Note 2)

Carry out all procedures at room temperature and employ aseptic techniques unless otherwise specified. Individuals who are immunocompromised or pregnant should not handle *L. monocytogenes*. The relevant institutional biosafety committee and animal facility management should be consulted before work commences.

3.1 Culturing and Long-Term Storage of L. monocytogenes

1. Dry HBA plates prior to use by pre-incubating at 37 °C overnight or placing uncovered in a laminar flow cabinet for 1 h (*see* **Notes 3** and **4**).
2. Obtain viable *L. monocytogenes* from one of the following: an infected mouse tissue homogenate, a lyophilized stock, a frozen glycerol stock (*see* **Note 5**), or a colony from a recent *L. monocytogenes* culture (*see* **Note 6**).
3. Streak *L. monocytogenes* on a HBA plate as shown in Fig. 1 using a sterile inoculating loop. Incubate at 37 °C overnight.
4. Pick a single colony from a fresh *L. monocytogenes* culture on a HBA plate using a sterilized inoculating loop and inoculate 10 mL of brain heart infusion (BHI) broth in a 30 mL McCartney bottle.
5. Incubate the *L. monocytogenes* culture in an orbital shaker at 180 rpm at 37 °C overnight.
6. Add sterile 80 % glycerol (v/v) to liquid *L. monocytogenes* BHI culture at a 1:1 ratio to obtain a final 40 % (v/v) glycerol concentration. Transfer 1 mL aliquots into cryovials and store at −70 °C.

3.2 Preparation and Storage of L. monocytogenes Infectious Stock for In Vivo Infection of Mice (See Note 7)

1. Streak *L. monocytogenes* from a frozen glycerol stock onto a HBA plate as shown in Fig. 1. Incubate plates at 37 °C overnight for use on the next day.
2. Pick a single *L. monocytogenes* colony from the cultured HBA plate and inoculate a 10 mL BHI broth. Avoid transferring agar into the broth.
3. Incubate the *L. monocytogenes* BHI culture in an orbital shaker at 180 rpm and 37 °C to mid-logarithmic phase, which typically has an optical density reading at 600 nm (OD600) of ~0.4. This typically takes 3–4 h; at which time, take a 0.9 mL aliquot aseptically for an OD600 reading. If the OD600 reading is <0.4, then continue to culture bacteria in an orbital shaker at 180 rpm and 37 °C until the OD600 reading is ~0.4.
4. Add 1 mL of sterile 80 % glycerol (v/v) to 10 mL of *L. monocytogenes* BHI broth culture (OD600 ~0.4). Mix gently and transfer into 1.5 mL microfuge tubes in 1 mL aliquots (*see* **Note 8**).
5. Place the aliquots on ice for 10 min and store at −70 °C (*see* **Note 9**). Leave one aliquot unfrozen to determine the concentration of *L. monocytogenes* in the infectious stock, which is typically in the order of 10^9 CFU/mL.
6. Perform 1:10 serial dilutions of the unfrozen *L. monocytogenes* infectious stock in PBS to 10^{-8} dilution. Spread 100 μL of undiluted and each subsequent dilution onto pre-dried HBA plates in duplicate, from the lowest to the highest concentration, using a sterile spreader. Incubate plates at 37 °C overnight.

7. Count the number of colonies on each plate and determine the *L. monocytogenes* concentration of the frozen infectious stock culture using the following calculation: concentration (CFU/mL) = number of colonies × dilution factor/0.1 mL. The plates chosen for counting should ideally have 30–300 colonies to ensure a reliable estimate of the CFU.
8. A few days after storing *L. monocytogenes* infectious stock at −70 °C, thaw out one tube. Determine the concentration of viable *L. monocytogenes* as described in **steps 6** and 7. This concentration should be similar to that determined for the freshly prepared infectious stock in **step 7** (*see* **Note 10**).

3.3 Optimization and Administration of Antibody for In Vivo Depletion of Immune Cell Subsets (See Note 11)

1. Obtain purified antibody that will specifically deplete the desired immune cell subset in *L. monocytogenes* infected mice (*see* **Note 12**).
2. Prepare different amounts of the depleting antibody stock in 400 μL of PBS to determine the effective dose for in vivo depletion of the chosen immune cell subset (*see* **Note 13**). Isotype-matching nonreactive antibodies, such as rat antibody, can be used as a control treatment.
3. Restrain the mouse to be injected by scruffing the back of the mouse and securing the mouse in an extended conformation with the abdomen of the mouse facing up for intraperitoneal injection. Clean the injection site with an 80 % ethanol wipe Insert the needle into the peritoneal cavity along the midline of the mouse with the needle pointing toward the mouse's head and as flat as possible to the mouse's body surface to avoid injecting the gastrointestinal tract. Inject 400 μL of the depleting antibody solution using a syringe with a 27 gauge needle. Observe that no bleeding occurs at the site of injection as the needle is drawn out of the mouse (bleeding may indicate an internal organ was accidentally damaged by the injection). Return the mouse to its cage.
4. Euthanize the treated mouse at the desired time point (*see* **Note 14**) after injection using a method approved by the local Animal Ethics Committee, such as CO_2 asphyxiation (*see* **Note 15**).
5. Perform a cardiac bleed immediately after euthanasia using a 1 mL syringe and 25 gauge needle. Collect as much blood as possible into lithium heparin-coated Vacutainer tubes and keep samples on ice or at 4 °C.
6. Remove the liver and spleen from the mouse's body cavity using asceptic technique, place in FACS buffer, and keep on ice.
7. To prepare single-cell suspensions for FACS analysis from peripheral blood, go to Protocol 3.6; for the liver, go to Protocol 3.7; and for spleen, go to Protocol 3.8. Single-cell suspensions can then be stained with fluorescently labeled

antibodies specific for the appropriate cell-surface markers and analyzed by flow cytometry to determine the optimal antibody dose required for cell depletion in vivo (*see* **Note 16**).

8. For in vivo depletion of immune cell subsets in mice infected with *L. monocytogenes*, determine if depletion should occur before or after bacteria injection (*see* **Note 17**).
9. If depletion is desired after injection with *L. monocytogenes*, then proceed to Protocol 3.4.
10. Prepare the optimal dose for the depleting antibody in 400 μL of PBS and intraperitoneally inject the antibody into the peritoneal cavity (*see* **Note 18**).

3.4 Preparation of L. monocytogenes Inoculum and Intravenous Injection of Mice

1. Determine the concentration of *L. monocytogenes* to be injected per mouse (*see* **Note 19**). For intravenous injection, mice receive a 200 μL inoculum.
2. Thaw out a frozen aliquot of *L. monocytogenes* infectious stock (from Protocol 3.2). Dilute the infectious stock in PBS to the desired *L. monocytogenes* concentration (*see* **Note 20**). Double the volume needed for injecting all mice to ensure that there is enough inoculum for both injection and determination of the *L. monocytogenes* CFU pre- and post-injection.
3. Remove 2× 0.1 mL aliquots from the prepared *L. monocytogenes* inoculum, and prepare serial 1:10 dilutions in PBS for each aliquot before injection of mice (*see* **Note 21**). Spread 0.1 mL of each dilution on HBA plates, and incubate the plates at 37 °C overnight. Count the number of colonies and determine the pre-injection concentration of the *L. monocytogenes* inoculum: concentration (CFU/mL) = (number of colonies × dilution factor)/mL plated for that dilution factor.
4. Transfer the mouse to be injected into a clean cage. Warm the mouse by placing the cage ~50 cm under a 250 W infrared lamp for 5 min (*see* **Note 22**). Place the mouse in a suitable restraining device for tail vein injections.
5. Gently mix the *L. monocytogenes* suspension to maintain a consistent suspension each time a syringe is loaded.
6. Locate the lateral tail vein of the mouse, gently wipe with an 80 % ethanol wipe and inject 200 μL of the *L. monocytogenes* inoculum (at the desired concentration) using a syringe with a 27 gauge needle into the tail vein. Briefly apply pressure to the entry wound with a sterile wipe. Return the mouse to its cage (*see* **Note 23**).
7. Once injection of all mice is completed and syringe(s) have been safely discarded, repeat **step 3** using the remaining amount of the inoculum to determine the post-injection concentration of the *L. monocytogenes* inoculum.

8. The amount of *L. monocytogenes* injected into mice is reported as the average CFU determined from the pre- and post-injection *L. monocytogenes* inoculum samples.
9. If depletion of a particular immune cell subset is desired at a certain time post-injection of *L. monocytogenes*, then proceed to Protocol 3.3 and *see* **Note 17**. If not, then proceed to Protocol 3.5.

3.5 Removal of Blood, Liver and Spleen from Infected Mice for Analyses

1. Euthuanize the infected mouse at the desired time point post-infection using a method approved by the local Animal Ethics Committee, such as CO_2 asphyxiation (*see* **Note 15**).
2. If peripheral blood is required, perform a cardiac bleed immediately after euthanasia using a 1 mL syringe and 25 gauge needle. Collect as much blood as possible into lithium heparin-coated Vacutainer tubes and store samples on ice or at 4 °C (go to Protocol 3.6 to prepare peripheral blood cell suspension for FACS analysis).
3. Remove the gall bladder and severe the inferior vena cava. Expose the hepatic portal vein by carefully pushing the intestines to the right. Flip the liver lobes toward the mouse's head and to the left so the liver is sitting where the diaphragm is located. The hepatic portal vein feeds into the bottom of the liver from the lower right hand side.
4. Perfuse the liver by injecting 10 mL of PBS into the hepatic portal vein using a 26 gauge needle bent at approximately 30° (*see* **Note 24**). PBS injected through the portal vein will exit from the severed inferior vena cava (*see* **Note 25**).
5. Remove the perfused liver from the mouse's body cavity, place in FACS buffer (*see* **Note 26**), and keep on ice. Go to Protocol 3.7 for the preparation of the liver for FACS analysis.
6. Remove the spleen from the mouse, place in FACS buffer, and store on ice.
7. Cut the spleen in half and weigh each half. Place one half in FACS buffer (*see* **Note 26**) and proceed to Protocol 3.8. Place the other half in a Stomacher bag on ice and go to Protocol 3.9.

3.6 Preparation of Peripheral Blood Cell Suspension for FACS Analysis

1. Measure and record the volume of blood taken to estimate the leukocyte concentration. Transfer blood into 5 mL of TAC buffer to lyse erythrocytes and incubate at room temperature for up to 10 min with frequent inversion. Collect cells by centrifugation at 230×*g* for 5 min at 4 °C, discard supernatant, resuspend cells in 5 mL of TAC buffer, and incubate at room temperature for 5 min.
2. Underlay the cell suspension with 1 mL of FCS/EDTA buffer. Centrifuge at 350×*g* for 5 min at 4 °C, discard the supernatant, and resuspend the cell pellet in 0.5 mL of FACS/EDTA buffer.

3. Dilute the cell suspension 1:5–1:20 in trypan blue cell staining solution depending on the cell concentration. Count viable leukocytes using a hemocytometer and determine the total viable cells based on hemocytometer specifications. Single-cell suspensions can then be labeled with antibodies specific for desired cell-surface markers and analyzed by FACS.

3.7 Preparation of Hepatic Cell Suspension for FACS Analysis

1. Generate single-cell suspensions by placing liver with FACS buffer in a 70 μm cell strainer that is inside a 60 mm petri dish. Push the tissue through the cell strainer using a 5 mL rubber-capped syringe plunger until a single-cell suspension is formed (*see* **Note 27**).
2. Transfer the hepatic single-cell suspension from the petri dish to a 50 mL conical screw-cap tube and bring the total volume to 40 mL with cold FACS buffer.
3. Vortex the cell suspension and, if necessary, take a 1 mL aliquot to determine the bacterial load for the liver. This 1 mL aliquot can be used in place of the tissue homogenate in the Stomacher bag described in Protocol 3.9.
4. Collect the cells by centrifugation at 500 × *g* for 5 min at 4 °C, discard the supernatant, and resuspend the cell pellet in 40 mL of cold FACS buffer. Repeat the centrifugation step at 500 × *g* for 5 min at 4 °C and discard supernatant.
5. Resuspend the cell pellet in 20 mL of isotonic Percoll at room temperature. Centrifuge the cell suspension at 700 × *g* for 12 min at room temperature. Discard the supernatant and disk-like sheet of cells that are floating on the top of the Percoll (i.e., hepatocytes). Resuspend the leukocyte-containing pellet in 4 mL of TAC buffer to lyse erythrocytes and incubate cells at room temperature for up to 10 min with frequent inversion.
6. Filter the cell suspension through a 100 μm nylon membrane into a new 10 mL centrifuge tube.
7. Underlay the filtered cell suspension with 1 mL of FCS/EDTA buffer. Centrifuge at 350 × *g* for 5 min at 4 °C. Discard the supernatant and resuspend the cell pellet in 5 mL of FACS/EDTA buffer.
8. Centrifuge the cell suspension at 350 × *g* for 5 min at 4 °C. Discard the supernatant and resuspend the cell pellet in 0.5–3 mL of FACS/EDTA buffer. The volume of buffer will depend on the size of the pellet.
9. Dilute the cell suspension 1:5–1:20 in trypan blue cell staining solution depending on the volume used to resuspend the cell pellet. Count the number of viable hepatic leukocytes using a hemocytometer. Hepatic single-cell suspensions can then be labeled with antibodies specific for desired cell-surface markers and analyzed by FACS (*see* Fig. 2 for representative example).

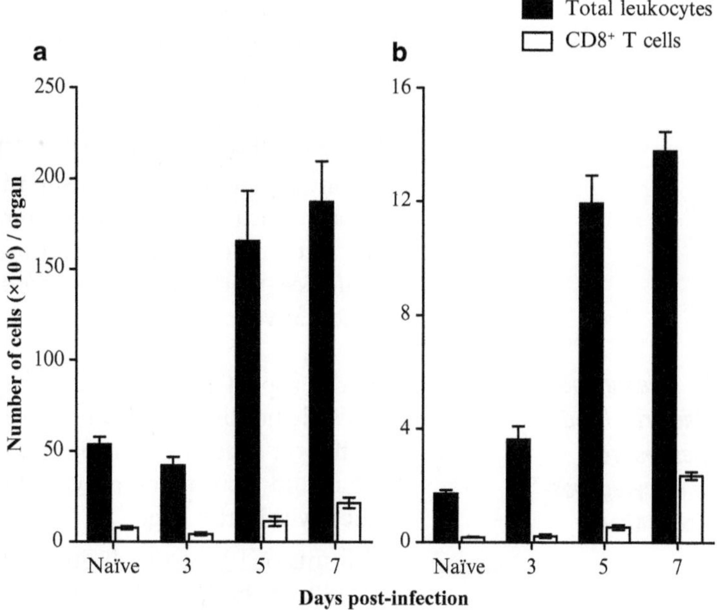

Fig. 2 FACS analysis of immune cells in *L. monocytogenes*-infected mice. Mice were infected with 1,000 CFU of *L. monocytogenes*. Single cell suspensions were prepared from the spleen (**a**) and liver (**b**) of naïve or infected mice at indicated time points post-infection. *Black columns* represent the mean total cellularity per organ, and *white columns* represent the mean number of $CD8^+$ T cells in each group. *Vertical bars* indicate standard error of mean. For each group and at each time point, at least five mice were analyzed

3.8 Preparation of Splenic Single-Cell Suspension for FACS Analysis

1. Generate a single-cell suspension by placing one half of the spleen with FACS buffer in a 70 μm cell strainer that is inside a 60 mm petri dish. Push the tissue through the cell strainer using a 5 mL rubber-capped syringe plunger until a single-cell suspension is formed (*see* **Note 27**).
2. Transfer the spleen single-cell suspension from the petri dish to a 10 mL centrifuge tube and bring the volume to 10 mL using cold FACS buffer.
3. Collect the cells by centrifugation at 500 × *g* for 5 min at 4 °C. Discard the supernatant and resuspend the cell pellet in 4 mL of TAC buffer to lyse eythrocytes. Incubate the cells at room temperature for up to 10 min with frequent inversion.
4. Filter the cell suspension through a 100 μm nylon membrane into a new 10 mL centrifuge tube.
5. Underlay the filtered cell suspension with 1 mL of FCS/EDTA buffer. Centrifuge at 350 × *g* for 5 min at 4 °C. Discard the supernatant and resuspend the cell pellet in 5 mL of FACS/ EDTA buffer.

6. Centrifuge the cell suspension at 350 × *g* for 5 min at 4 °C. Discard the supernatant and resuspend the cell pellet in 3–8 mL of FACS/EDTA buffer. The volume of buffer will depend on the size of the pellet.
7. Dilute the cell suspension 1:10–1:20 in trypan blue cell staining solution depending on resuspension volume. Count viable splenocytes using a hemocytometer. Splenic single-cell suspensions can then be labeled with antibodies specific for the desired cell-surface markers and analyzed by FACS (*see* Fig. 2 for representative example).

3.9 Measurement of Bacterial Load in Tissues from *L. monocytogenes*-Infected Mice

1. Fold the top of the Stomacher bag containing the spleen in half. While holding the Stomacher bag shut to prevent leakage, lay it flat on a clean bench or in a laminar flow cabinet. Roll a thick round pen/marker over the tissue until the tissue is mashed within the bag.
2. Add 5 mL of PBS to each Stomacher bag containing mashed tissue. Place the Stomacher bag into the Stomacher, and run the Stomacher on high speed for 10 min (*see* **Note 28**).
3. Mix the homogenate in the Stomacher bag (or the 1 mL aliquot of hepatic cell suspension from Protocol 3.7) with a pipette. Transfer 300 μL to a 96-well flat bottom plate. Within the wells of the 96-well plate perform 1:10 serial dilutions (30 μL into 270 μL PBS) to a 10^{-5} dilution for each tissue homogenate sample. Perform the serial dilutions in duplicates for each sample.
4. Carefully spread 0.1 mL of each dilution onto a pre-dried HBA plate using a sterile or re-sterilized spreader from the lowest to highest concentration (*see* **Note 29**). Incubate plates at 37 °C overnight (or at room temperature for 2–3 days).
5. Count the number of CFU for each dilution plate (*see* **Notes 30** and **31**) and calculate the CFU per tissue taking into account the portion of the tissue (e.g., half a spleen), dilution factor, and the total volume of tissue homogenate (5 mL or 40 mL): CFU/tissue = CFU/0.1 mL × dilution factor × mL/tissue; for spleen divide this number by the percentage weight of the spleen sample used for tissue homogenization (*see* Fig. 3 for representative example).

4 Notes

1. Susceptibility to *L. monocytogenes* infection varies between mouse strains [31].
2. A video demonstrating some of the methods and techniques described in this chapter can be found at www.jove.com/video/3076/ [33].

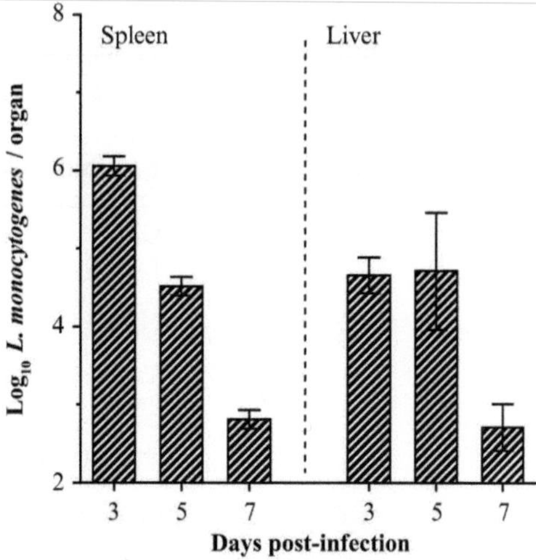

Fig. 3 *L. monocytogenes* infection kinetics in the spleen and liver. Mice were infected with 1,000 CFU of *L. monocytogenes*. The bacterial load was determined at the indicated time points post-infection. At each time point, $n=5$, and the geometric mean ± standard error is shown

3. Growth of *L. monocytogenes* can be supported on different nonselective media, such as a range of blood agar (supplemented with horse, sheep, guinea pig or human blood brain heart infusion (BHI) agar or broth, or tryptic soy broth with yeast extract (TSB-YE)). Alternatively, Oxford formulation media can be used. This formulation is high in salinity and selectively supports the growth of *L. monocytogenes*, while minimizing the growth of other bacteria.
4. Drying the HBA plates ensures that there is optimal separation of bacterial colonies on the plate.
5. When deriving fresh *L. monocytogenes* cultures from a frozen glycerol stock, the first passage should be made on agar plates because *L. monocytogenes* obtained from frozen glycerol stocks grow poorly when directly subcultured in liquid medium.
6. When using *L. monocytogenes* from a recent culture, the culture should be less than one-week old and not subcultured more than 10 generations.
7. Although initially more time consuming than preparing a fresh *L. monocytogenes* inoculum for a single experiment, preparing frozen *L. monocytogenes* infectious stocks enables accurate determination of the CFU concentration prior to infection and improves consistency between experiments when mice are infected from the same batch of frozen stock.
8. *L. monocytogenes* inoculum is frozen at a lower percentage glycerol (8 %) than for *L. monocytogenes* frozen for general long-term storage (40 %).

Table 1
Antibodies used for the depletion of immune cell subsets in previous reports of mice infected with *L. monocytogenes*

Cell type	Targeted antigen	Antibody clone	Reference
Neutrophils	Gr-1 Ly-6G	RB6-8C5 1A8	[21, 22] [34, 35]
NK cells	NK1.1	PK136	[36]
γδ-T cells	TCR γδ chain	UC7-13D5 GL3	[37, 38] [39, 40]
αβ-T cells	TCR β chain	H57-597	[37, 39, 40]
$CD4^+$ T cells	CD4 (L3T4)	GK1.5	[41, 42]
$CD8^+$ T cells	CD8	2.43 53-6.7	[43] [44, 45]
B cells	CD20	MB20-11	[46]

9. Frozen *L. monocytogenes* infectious stocks are typically stable at −70 °C for up to 6 months.
10. If the concentration of the thawed *L. monocytogenes* infectious stock exhibits a >20 % decline in CFU compared to the freshly prepared stock, then a new frozen infectious stock should be prepared.
11. Skip to Protocol 3.4 if it is not desired to determine the effect of depleting an immune cell subset upon bacterial load and/or immune responses in *L. monocytogenes* infected mice.
12. *See* Table 1 for a list of antibodies that have previously been reported to deplete immune cell subsets. We recommend using commercially purchased antibody that has been purified and free of antibiotics. If produced "in-house", then ensure that the antibody preparation is free of contaminating antibiotics and other chemicals.
13. Even if a recommended dose is provided for the depleting antibody, it is best to confirm this dose in the appropriate in vivo model. We typically test the following amounts in 400 μL of PBS: 0.0, 0.1, 0.2, 0.5, 1.0 mg. If cell depletion is to occur post-infection, then the optimal antibody dose for cell depletion should be determined using *L. monocytogenes*-infected mice (as in Fig. 4).
14. To determine the time period for the depletion effect, different time points should be tested post-injection of the depleting antibody (e.g., 24, 48, 72 h).

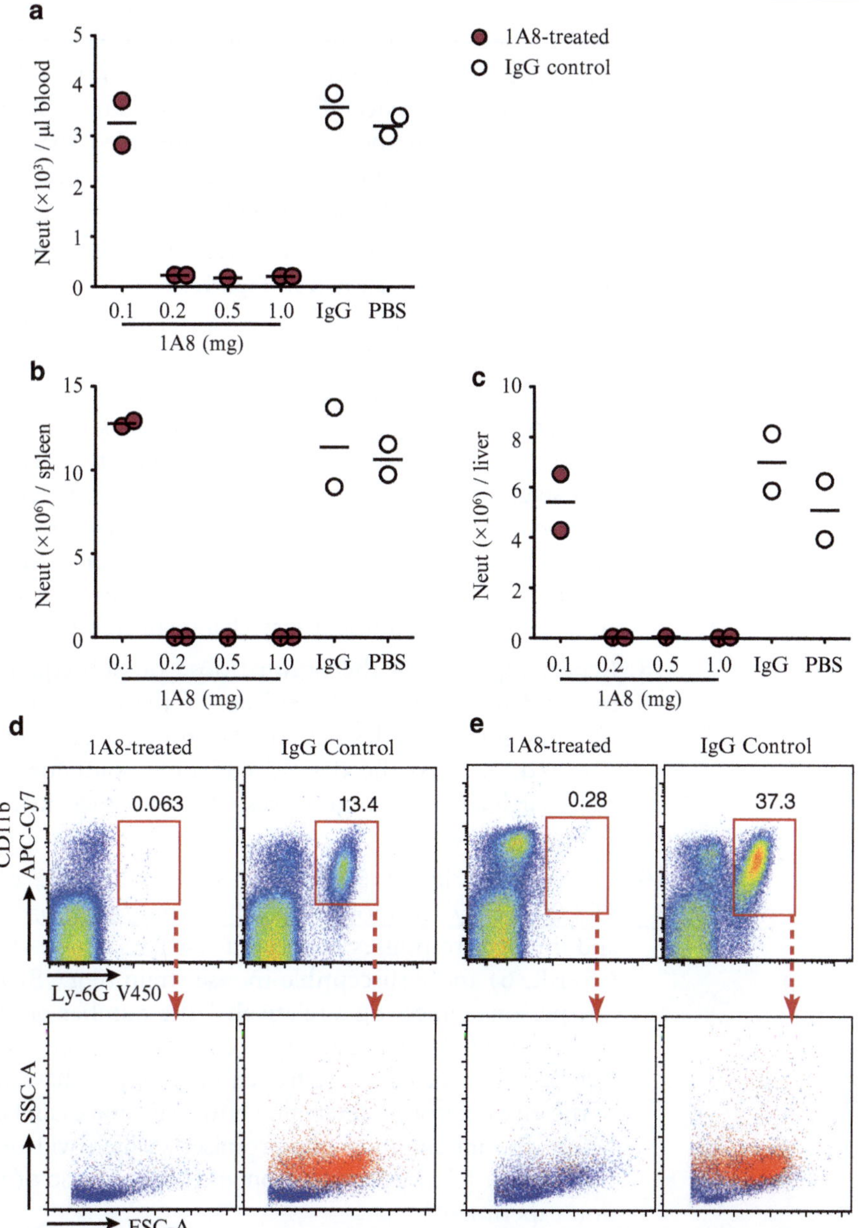

Fig. 4 Treatment optimization for neutrophil depletion in mice using a neutrophil-specific antibody (1A8). Mice were infected with 1,000 CFU of *L. monocytogenes*. Neutrophil-depleting antibody (1A8) was intraperitoneally administered at the indicated dose at day 2 post-infection. The number of neutrophils in the blood (**a**), spleen (**b**), and liver (**c**) was determined by flow cytometry 24 h after antibody injection. Representative FACS plots indicate that the injection of 1A8, but not IgG control antibody, successfully depleted $CD11b^{+}Ly6G^{+}$ cells (i.e., neutrophils) from the spleen (**d**) and liver (**e**). *Note*: Where possible, employ antibodies with specificity for different epitopes on the same cell markers to confirm depletion efficiency of the desired cell subset

15. For euthanasia of mice, CO_2 asphyxiation is the preferred method because it has minimal impact on bacterial CFU and immune cell viability in the spleen and liver. If blood collection is not required, cervical dislocation may be used as an alternative euthanasia method. It is recommended that euthanasia methods not be used that may affect organ weight or immune cell viability (e.g., thiobarbiturates).
16. An example of optimizing the 1A8 antibody for neutrophil depletion in mice is shown in Fig. 4.
17. Depletion of immune cells prior to injection of *L. monocytogenes* enables assessment of early immune responses and bacterial load in the absence of the depleted immune cell subset. Alternatively, depletion of immune cells at different times post-injection of *L. monocytogenes* enables assessment of immune cells during the later stages of infection and bacterial clearance. If cell-depletion is to be induced post-injection of *L. monocytogenes,* it is recommended that the effective antibody dose be determined in infected mice, rather than naïve mice, because the cell number and/or rate of recruitment may change in an infectious setting.
18. Repeat injection of the optimal dose on subsequent days as required based on (1) the efficacy of the depleting antibody, (2) how long it is desired for the immune cell subset to be depleted, and (3) the desired end time-point for analysis of bacterial load and immune responses in mice infected with *L. monocytogenes.*
19. We typically inject 500–3,000 CFU (200 μL of 2,500–15,000 CFU/mL inoculum) when comparing bacterial load and immune responses between a resistant mouse strain (e.g., C57BL/6) and a susceptible mouse strain (e.g., BALB/c). If one person is injecting a relatively large number of mice, then the *L. monocytogenes* viability (i.e., CFU concentration) may reduce over time once the frozen inoculum is thawed. It is up to the investigator to determine how many mice can be injected before the inoculum is compromised, which will depend on the starting CFU concentration and the purpose of the infection experiment.
20. If the infectious stock will not be diluted in PBS by at least 10^5, then a washing step should be added to remove residual media/glycerol as follows: Add 9 mL of PBS to thawed infectious stock and bacteria collected by centrifugation at 2,100 × *g* for 10 min at 4 °C. Remove the supernatant and resuspend the pelleted bacterial cells in 10 mL of sterile PBS. Repeat the centrifugation and resuspend the bacteria cell pellet in the desired volume. It should be noted that a washing step may result in some loss of bacteria. It is also recommended that such loss be

determined beforehand and accounted for diluting the inoculum to the required concentration.

21. If the desired CFU concentration for the inoculum is high, then be sure to perform 1:10 serial dilutions to ensure an accurate determination of the CFU concentration (i.e., the inoculums should be diluted such that single colonies can be easily distinguished and counted on the HBA plate, ideally at 30–300 colonies per plate).
22. Other suitable thermal devices that will not burn the mouse or increase the temperature of the cage above 40 °C can also be used.
23. We observe that mice infected with sublethal doses of *L. monocytogenes* using this protocol may transiently exhibit ruffled fur, hunched posture, and weight loss within the first few days. These symptoms provide a visual cue based on how severely an individual mouse is affected by the infection, whether it responds differently to the rest of the group (i.e., an "obvious" outlier), and whether euthanasia is necessary to prevent excessive suffering and impending death due to the infection.
24. A ½ in. length 26 gauge needle that is bent by ~30° can better facilitate injection of PBS into the hepatic portal vein.
25. When perfused properly, the liver turns from a dark red color to light brown after injecting 1–2 mL of PBS. Liver perfusion ensures that harvested cells are from the liver and not the circulating blood. If the liver is not required for FACS analysis, perfusion is not necessary. The liver can be isolated and collected directly into a Stomacher bag and processed as described for the spleen in Protocol 3.9.
26. Use sufficient FACS buffer to completely submerge the tissue to minimize the exposure of any part of the tissue to air.
27. Keep cells on ice unless otherwise specified.
28. If a Stomacher is not available, a tissue homogenizer can be used instead. Alternatively, the following method, although not as efficient, can also be used to manually macerate the organ: place the organ in a sealed sterilized plastic bag and lay on a clean bench while holding the bag shut to prevent leakage; roll a 500 mL laboratory glass bottle repeatedly over the bag until the tissue is thoroughly mashed; and add 5 mL of PBS to each bag.
29. It is important that the HBA plate be dried thoroughly (i.e., no moisture on the agar). Otherwise it may be difficult to obtain distinct *L. monocytogenes* colonies that can be counted properly.
30. There should be a clear reduction in the number of colonies as the dilution factor becomes higher, such that counting distinct CFU is possible for at least one dilution. If the mouse has

cleared the *L. monocytogenes* infection (i.e., detection limit = 100 CFU/tissue), then <5 *L. monocytogenes* colonies will be present on the HBA plate that was spread with 0.2 mL of the undiluted homogenate. To more accurately measure lower values for CFU/organ, a larger amount of the tissue homogenate can be cultured (up to 0.5 mL per plate) so a greater proportion of tissue is sampled for detection of *L. monocytogenes*.

31. If the liver and/or spleen become contaminated with intestinal or other external bacteria during isolation, the colonies on the HBA plate are likely to exhibit different morphology (i.e., they will not have the characteristic halo and pale color of *Listeria* colonies) and/or may be different in colony counts to what is expected for *L. monocytogenes* (i.e., too few or too many).

Acknowledgments

The authors would like to thank Anna Walduck, Christina Cheers, Patrick Reading, Andrew Brooks, Stuart Berzins, Dale Godfrey, Yifan Zhan, and Jonathan Wilksch for advice and reagents. This work was supported by the Juvenile diabetes Research Foundation (1-2008-602), the Australian National Health and Medical Research Council (1029231, 1030865), and the Victorian Government's Operational Infrastructure Support Program. NW is supported by an Australian Postgraduate Award. O.L.W. is supported by a RD Wright Fellowship from the Australian National Health and Medical Research Council.

References

1. Pamer EG (2004) Immune responses to *Listeria monocytogenes*. Nat Rev Immunol 4:812–823
2. Garifulin O, Boyartchuk V (2005) *Listeria monocytogenes* as a probe of immune function. Brief Funct Genomic Proteomic 4:258–269
3. Cossart P (2011) Illuminating the landscape of host-pathogen interactions with the bacterium *Listeria monocytogenes*. Proc Natl Acad Sci U S A 108:19484–19491
4. Unanue ER, Carrero JA (2012) Studies with *Listeria monocytogenes* lead the way. Adv Immunol 113:1–5
5. Wing EJ, Gregory SH (2002) *Listeria monocytogenes*: clinical and experimental update. J Infect Dis 185(Suppl 1):S18–S24
6. Conlan JW (1999) Early host-pathogen interactions in the liver and spleen during systemic murine listeriosis: an overview. Immunobiology 201:178–187
7. Cousens LP, Wing EJ (2000) Innate defenses in the liver during *Listeria* infection. Immunol Rev 174:150–159
8. den Bakker HC, Cummings CA, Ferreira V, Vatta P, Orsi RH, Degoricija L, Barker M, Petrauskene O, Furtado MR, Wiedmann M (2010) Comparative genomics of the bacterial genus *Listeria*: genome evolution is characterized by limited gene acquisition and limited gene loss. BMC Genomics 11:688
9. Lara-Tejero M, Pamer EG (2004) T cell responses to *Listeria monocytogenes*. Curr Opin Microbiol 7:45–50
10. Portnoy DA, Auerbuch V, Glomski IJ (2002) The cell biology of *Listeria monocytogenes* infection: the intersection of bacterial pathogenesis and cell-mediated immunity. J Cell Biol 158:409–414
11. Condotta SA, Richer MJ, Badovinac VP, Harty JT (2012) Probing CD8 T cell responses with

Listeria monocytogenes infection. Adv Immunol 113:51–80

12. Serbina NV, Shi C, Pamer EG (2012) Monocyte-mediated immune defense against murine Listeria monocytogenes infection. Adv Immunol 113:119–134
13. Witte CE, Archer KA, Rae CS, Sauer JD, Woodward JJ, Portnoy DA (2012) Innate immune pathways triggered by *Listeria monocytogenes* and their role in the induction of cell-mediated immunity. Adv Immunol 113:135–156
14. Lam GY, Czuczman MA, Higgins DE, Brumell JH (2012) Interactions of *Listeria monocytogenes* with the autophagy system of host cells. Adv Immunol 113:7–18
15. Edelson BT (2012) Dendritic cells in Listeria monocytogenes infection. Adv Immunol 113:33–49
16. Carrero JA, Unanue ER (2012) Mechanisms and immunological effects of apoptosis caused by *Listeria monocytogenes*. Adv Immunol 113: 157–174
17. Busch DH, Vijh S, Pamer EG (2001) Animal model for infection with *Listeria monocytogenes*. Curr Protoc Immunol Chapter 19:Unit 19.9:1–9
18. Neuenhahn M, Schiemann M, Busch DH (2010) DCs in mouse models of intracellular bacterial infection. Methods Mol Biol 595:319–329
19. Gervais F, Stevenson M, Skamene E (1984) Genetic control of resistance to *Listeria monocytogenes*: regulation of leukocyte inflammatory responses by the Hc locus. J Immunol 132:2078–2083
20. Gervais F, Desforges C, Skamene E (1989) The C5-sufficient A/J congenic mouse strain. Inflammatory response and resistance to *Listeria monocytogenes*. J Immunol 142: 2057–2060
21. Conlan JW, North RJ (1994) Neutrophils are essential for early anti-*Listeria* defense in the liver, but not in the spleen or peritoneal cavity, as revealed by a granulocyte-depleting monoclonal antibody. J Exp Med 179:259–268
22. Czuprynski CJ, Brown JF, Wagner RD, Steinberg H (1994) Administration of anti-granulocyte monoclonal antibody RB6-8C5 prevents expression of acquired resistance to *Listeria monocytogenes* infection in previously immunized mice. Infect Immun 62: 5161–5163
23. Boyartchuk VL, Broman KW, Mosher RE, D'Orazio SE, Starnbach MN, Dietrich WF (2001) Multigenic control of *Listeria monocytogenes* susceptibility in mice. Nat Genet 27: 259–260
24. Boyartchuk V, Rojas M, Yan BS, Jobe O, Hurt N, Dorfman DM, Higgins DE, Dietrich WF, Kramnik I (2004) The host resistance locus sst1 controls innate immunity to *Listeria monocytogenes* infection in immunodeficient mice. J Immunol 173:5112–5120
25. Garifulin O, Qi Z, Shen H, Patnala S, Green MR, Boyartchuk V (2007) Irf3 polymorphism alters induction of interferon beta in response to *Listeria monocytogenes* infection. PLoS Genet 3:1587–1597
26. Cossart P, Toledo-Arana A (2008) *Listeria monocytogenes*, a unique model in infection biology: an overview. Microbes Infect 10:1041–1050
27. Mostowy S, Cossart P (2012) Virulence factors that modulate the cell biology of *Listeria* infection and the host response. Adv Immunol 113:19–32
28. Bruhn KW, Craft N, Miller JF (2007) *Listeria* as a vaccine vector. Microbes Infect 9:1226–1235
29. Guirnalda P, Wood L, Paterson Y (2012) *Listeria monocytogenes* and its products as agents for cancer immunotherapy. Adv Immunol 113:81–118
30. Lorber B (1997) Listeriosis. Clin Infect Dis 24:1–9
31. Cheers C, McKenzie IF (1978) Resistance and susceptibility of mice to bacterial infection: genetics of listeriosis. Infect Immun 19:755–762
32. Curtis GDW, Nichols WW, Falla TJ (1989) Selective agents for *Listeria* can inhibit their growth. Lett Appl Microbiol 8:169–172
33. Wang N, Strugnell R, Wijburg O, Brodnicki T (2011) Measuring bacterial load and immune responses in mice infected with Listeria monocytogenes. J Vis Exp 54:e3076. doi:10.3791/3076
34. Carr KD, Sieve AN, Indramohan M, Break TJ, Lee S, Berg RE (2011) Specific depletion reveals a novel role for neutrophil-mediated protection in the liver during *Listeria monocytogenes* infection. Eur J Immunol 41:2666–2676
35. Shi C, Hohl TM, Leiner I, Equinda MJ, Fan X, Pamer EG (2011) Ly6G+ neutrophils are dispensable for defense against systemic *Listeria monocytogenes* infection. J Immunol 187:5293–5298
36. Dunn PL, North RJ (1991) Early gamma interferon production by natural killer cells is important in defense against murine listeriosis. Infect Immun 59:2892–2900
37. Hiromatsu K, Yoshikai Y, Matsuzaki G, Ohga S, Muramori K, Matsumoto K, Bluestone JA, Nomoto K (1992) A protective role of gamma/delta T cells in primary infection with *Listeria monocytogenes* in mice. J Exp Med 175:49–56
38. Usami J, Hiromatsu K, Matsumoto Y, Maeda K, Inagaki H, Suzuki T, Yoshikai Y (1995) A protective role of gamma delta T cells in primary infection with *Listeria monocytogenes* in

autoimmune non-obese diabetic mice. Immunology 86:199–205
39. Skeen MJ, Ziegler HK (1993) Intercellular interactions and cytokine responsiveness of peritoneal alpha/beta and gamma/delta T cells from *Listeria*-infected mice: synergistic effects of interleukin 1 and 7 on gamma/delta T cells. J Exp Med 178:985–996
40. Fu YX, Roark CE, Kelly K, Drevets D, Campbell P, O'Brien R, Born W (1994) Immune protection and control of inflammatory tissue necrosis by gamma delta T cells. J Immunol 153:3101–3115
41. Shedlock DJ, Shen H (2003) Requirement for CD4 T cell help in generating functional CD8 T cell memory. Science 300:337–339
42. Sun JC, Bevan MJ (2003) Defective CD8 T cell memory following acute infection without CD4 T cell help. Science 300:339–342
43. Badovinac VP, Harty JT (2000) Adaptive immunity and enhanced CD8+ T cell response to *Listeria monocytogenes* in the absence of perforin and IFN-gamma. J Immunol 164: 6444–6452
44. Lukacs K, Kurlander R (1989) Lyt-2+ T cell-mediated protection against listeriosis. Protection correlates with phagocyte depletion but not with IFN-gamma production. J Immunol 142:2879–2886
45. Lauvau G, Vijh S, Kong P, Horng T, Kerksiek K, Serbina N, Tuma RA, Pamer EG (2001) Priming of memory but not effector CD8 T cells by a killed bacterial vaccine. Science 294:1735–1739
46. Bouaziz JD, Yanaba K, Venturi GM, Wang Y, Tisch RM, Poe JC, Tedder TF (2007) Therapeutic B cell depletion impairs adaptive and autoreactive CD4+ T cell activation in mice. Proc Natl Acad Sci U S A 104:20878–20883

Chapter 17

Mouse Model of Invasive Fungal Infection

Donna M. MacCallum

Abstract

The mouse intravenous (IV) challenge model of *Candida albicans* invasive fungal infection has been widely used to study the importance of the innate immune system in these infections. This chapter describes this well-characterized model, where fungal cells are administered directly into the mouse bloodstream to initiate a systemic infection. The preparation of tissue samples from infected mice to allow evaluation of disease progression and host responses is also described.

Key words Intravenous, Infection, *Candida albicans*, Virulence, Organ-specific, Immunity

1 Introduction

Although fungi are ubiquitous in the environment and are part of the natural flora of the human body, they can also cause a wide range of infections in susceptible humans. The most serious fungal infections are invasive or disseminated infections, which continue to have high mortality rates [1–4]. The major fungal species associated with invasive fungal infections are *Candida* species, particularly *Candida albicans*, with *Aspergillus* species common in certain patient groups. Invasive fungal infections are generally opportunistic, with innate immunity playing a major role in protection against these infections. The importance of the innate immune system is particularly obvious when risk factors for invasive fungal infection are investigated. *Candida* invasive infections are most common in patients who have resided in the Intensive Care Unit for more than 7 days, have been treated with broad spectrum antibiotics, are immunosuppressed (including neutropenic) and have experienced abdominal surgery (including solid organ transplant) or gut injury [2–5]. Invasive *Aspergillus* infections are mainly associated with hematological malignancies and stem cell transplants [1, 6–8].

Difficulties in diagnosis of invasive fungal infections, due to nonspecific symptoms [9–11], have made animal models essential for understanding the role of the innate immune system in these

Irving C. Allen (ed.), *Mouse Models of Innate Immunity: Methods and Protocols*, Methods in Molecular Biology, vol. 1031, DOI 10.1007/978-1-62703-481-4_17, © Springer Science+Business Media, LLC 2013

infections [12, 13]. Although other organisms have been used to model invasive fungal infections, mouse models remain the most commonly used due to cost, availability of reagents and knockout strains, as well as reproducibility of the model [12].

This chapter will describe the mouse intravenous (IV) challenge model of invasive fungal infection, which is commonly used to investigate innate immune responses that occur during these infections. In this model, fungal cells are administered directly into the mouse bloodstream and are rapidly dispersed throughout the animal [14, 15]. For *C. albicans* infections, the innate immune response rapidly clears fungal cells from most organs, but a delayed response in the kidneys allows infection to progress [16]. Disease progression in mice can be monitored by weight loss and increasing organ fungal burdens [14–16]. This is accompanied by increasing renal cytokine production, and eventually sepsis and death [14, 17–20]. Issues surrounding the use of different *C. albicans* strains/isolates and mouse strains, as well as various downstream analyses for mouse samples post-infection, are also discussed. Although this chapter concentrates on modelling invasive *C. albicans* infection, the principles are the same for intravenous infection with other pathogenic fungi.

2 Materials

2.1 Candida albicans Inoculum Preparation

1. *C. albicans* clinical isolates/laboratory strains (*see* **Note 1**).
2. YPD medium: 1 % (w/v) yeast extract, 2 % (w/v) mycological peptone, and 2 % (w/v) glucose.
3. Sabouraud agar plates: 1 % (w/v) mycological peptone, 4 % (w/v) glucose, and 2 % (w/v) agar.
4. NGY medium: 0.1 % (w/v) Neopeptone, 0.4 % (w/v) glucose, and 0.1 % (w/v) yeast extract (*see* **Note 2**).
5. Wire inoculation loop or disposable plastic inoculation loops.
6. Sterile physiological saline (*see* **Note 3**).
7. Neubauer hemocytometer.

2.2 Infection of Experimental Animals

1. Female BALB/c mice, 6–8 weeks old (specific pathogen-free) (Harlan) (*see* **Notes 4–9**).
2. Weighing balance.
3. Heat lamp or warm box (*see* **Note 10**).
4. Mouse restraining device (*see* **Note 11**).
5. 26G or 27G syringe needles (*see* **Note 12**).
6. 1 mL Leur-Lok syringes.
7. Tissues/cotton wool.

2.3 Assessing Experimental Infection and Innate Immune Response

1. Blunt-ended microcentrifuge tubes (2 mL) containing 0.5 mL of sterile physiological saline (optional: protease inhibitors added to saline) (weights recorded).
2. 70 % ethanol.
3. Sterile scissors and forceps.
4. CAT homogenizer (model: X1030D) and dispersal tool.
5. Multiplex cytokine immunoassays e.g., cytometric bead arrays (BD Biosciences) or Bio-Plex assays (Biorad).

3 Methods

3.1 Planning

1. The investigator must ensure that they have the necessary permissions and/or licenses required for studies involving animals (*see* **Note 13**).
2. Calculate the number of animals per experimental group. This depends upon the variation observed between experimental animals (which can depend upon the skill and experience of the researcher), as well as the level of difference expected between control and experimental groups. Using the well-established *C. albicans* i.v. challenge model in female BALB/c mice, we rarely require more than 6 animals per group.
3. Clearly define experimental end points and plan for the samples required for downstream analyses. Experimental end points can be predetermined sampling time points or may rely upon identification of severely ill animals. Researchers should be able to recognize severe illness in mice which includes the following symptoms: hunched posture; ruffled coat; weight loss; immobility; and decreased body temperature. Mice should be humanely terminated (*see* **Note 14**) when they show signs of severe illness.

3.2 C. albicans Inocula

1. Retrieve *C. albicans* isolates/strains from −80 °C freezer stocks and grow on Sabouraud or YPD agar at 30 °C.
2. Prepare a culture for inoculum. Using an inoculation loop, touch the surface of a single colony on the agar plate, then aseptically inoculate a sterile glass test tube containing 5 mL of NGY medium. Repeat for all *C. albicans* strains/isolates to be tested.
3. Incubate the tubes in a rotating wheel at 30 °C for 16–24 h.
4. Harvest the cultures by centrifugation and wash twice with sterile physiological saline. Resuspend washed cells in sterile physiological saline and determine the cell concentration using a Neubauer hemocytometer. Dilute the cell suspension with sterile physiological saline to obtain the desired cell concentration (*see* **Note 15**).

5. Confirm the actual inoculum level by spotting aliquots of serial dilutions (1:10) of the inoculum on Sabouraud agar plates and incubating the plates overnight at 35 °C. Count the colony forming units (CFU) for each dilution and then calculate the CFU per mL for the neat inoculum. Calculate the actual inoculum as CFU/g mouse body weight as follows: multiply by the volume (in mL) injected and then divide by the mouse weight (in g).
6. Transport inocula to the animal facility in packaging which satisfies local rules regarding transport of biosafety level 2/hazard group 2 and/or genetically modified organisms (if applicable).

3.3 Intravenous Infection of Mice

1. One day prior to infection, randomly allocate female BALB/c mice into experimental groups. Mark mice to allow identification and monitoring of individual animals, and record individual weights prior to infection.
2. Heat mice to allow clear visualization of the lateral tail veins (*see* **Note 16**).
3. Prior to infection, invert the inocula to mix. Load 1 mL syringes, taking care to remove all air bubbles from the syringe (*see* **Note 17**).
4. Place a mouse in the restraining device. Hold the tail firmly to prevent the mouse from moving, but not too tightly as this will restrict blood flow. Locate the lateral tail veins by gently turning the tail 90°. The lateral tail veins should be obvious in albino mice.
5. Bend the mouse tail over one finger and gently insert the syringe needle into a lateral tail vein. The tail vein is just below the surface of the tail. In BALB/c mice, and other albino mouse strains, the needle should remain visible even when within the vein. There should be no resistance as the needle enters the vein.
6. Gently depress the syringe plunger to dispense the correct volume. Again, there should be no resistance. Any resistance or evidence of whitening and/or swelling suggests that the needle is not in the correct position. A successful injection is indicated by the vein lightening as the inoculum is dispensed, and then filling again with blood.
7. In the case of an unsuccessful injection, a second attempt should be made using either the other lateral tail vein or another spot closer to the base of the tail in the same vein.
8. Stop any bleeding by holding a tissue or cotton wool ball over the injection spot for a short time. Return mice to their cage.
9. Monitor mice for at least 5 min post-injection for signs of adverse reactions.

3.4 Daily Mouse Monitoring

1. Check the mice at least once daily post-infection. Evaluate mouse condition and record individual mouse weights. Weight loss is a good indicator of disease progression, with 20 % weight loss predictive of imminent death in BALB/c mice [14]. Mice losing 20 % of their initial body weight should be humanely terminated (e.g., by terminal anesthesia, cervical dislocation or CO_2 asphyxiation) (*see* **Note 14**). Death is recorded as having occurred on the following day.

3.5 Sampling and Evaluating Fungal Infection and Host Responses

1. At the time of death or at predetermined time points, terminate animals by cervical dislocation or terminal anesthesia. Spray carcasses with 70 % ethanol and dissect the organs of interest with aseptic precautions. In *C. albicans* invasive fungal infections, the kidneys are sampled as this is the organ where *C. albicans* infection progresses.

   Harvested organs yield valuable information, such as fungal burden, cytokine/chemokine profiles, histological changes, immune cell population analysis, and RNA for gene expression analyses.
2. To determine organ fungal burdens, weigh the organs and homogenize in 0.5 mL of saline. Plate dilutions of the organ homogenate on Sabouraud agar and incubate overnight at 35 °C. The next day count the colonies, and then calculate fungal CFU per mL homogenate. Express fungal burdens per gram of tissue by dividing the fungal CFU/mL by the weight of tissue per mL homogenate.
3. For cytokine analyses, homogenize mouse organs in saline with added protease inhibitors to prevent degradation of cytokines during storage. Centrifuge the homogenized tubes at full speed in a chilled benchtop centrifuge to remove cell debris. Transfer the supernatant into a fresh tube and store at −20 °C until ready to analyze using a multiplex kit. These kits allow multiple cytokines to be measured in a single reaction. Alternatively, ELISAs can be carried out; however, the amount of supernatant obtained per sample is often a limiting factor.
4. For histological analyses, preserve tissue pieces in either formalin (for paraffin wax-embedding) or in OCT with subsequent flash-freezing in liquid nitrogen (for frozen sections). Cut 8 μm sections on a microtome (paraffin blocks) or with a cryostat (frozen blocks) and then stain as required to visualize fungi, organ structures and/or immune infiltrates. Fungi can be clearly visualized by periodic acid Schiff staining or by Grocott's silver staining.
5. For RNA extraction and subsequent analysis of gene expression, flash-freeze pieces of tissue in liquid nitrogen or dispense droplets of organ homogenates into liquid nitrogen. Allow the liquid nitrogen to evaporate and store frozen material at −80 °C until ready to extract RNA using Trizol reagent.

4 Notes

1. In the mouse i.v. challenge model, *C. albicans* clinical isolates show variation in virulence [21, 22]. Laboratory strains, used in the creation of genetically modified strains, can also have altered virulence, which may be due to chromosomal aneuploidies [23]. Therefore, the behavior of the chosen isolate or strain should initially be characterized in a small pilot study.
2. We routinely use NGY medium to prepare inocula for mouse infection, as this medium gives reproducible cell numbers per mL when *C. albicans* is grown under our standard conditions and there is little evidence of filamentous growth. Other growth media can be used, but it should be remembered that *C. albicans* virulence is altered when the fungus is grown in different media [24].
3. Fungal cells for i.v. administration are suspended in sterile physiological saline intended for administration to human patients. This has the added advantage, from an immunological point of view, of being pyrogen-free.
4. A number of different mouse strains, including outbred and inbred strains, have been used in *C. albicans* i.v. challenge models of infection. Inbred mouse strains show less biological variation between individual animals; however, different mouse strains vary considerably in their susceptibility to *C. albicans* i.v. infection, with A/J and DBA/2 (complement C5 deficient) mice being much more susceptible to *C. albicans* i.v. infection [25–27].

   The choice of mouse strain may also be dictated if knockout mouse strains are to be used. The majority of knockout mouse strains have been created in a C57BL/6 background. This significantly affects the ease with which injections are performed. Albino (e.g., BALB/c and CD-1) mouse strains have no pigment in their tails, allowing tail veins to be more easily visualized. In contrast, black mice, such as C57BL/6, have pigmented tails which makes it much more difficult to distinguish the tail veins. For investigators with little experience performing i.v. injections, it is recommended that initial experiments be performed in albino mice whenever possible.
5. Mice purchased from a commercial supplier should be allowed an adjustment period of 5–7 days prior to any experimentation being performed.
6. In immunological studies the use of specific pathogen-free mice is particularly important as mice infected with other pathogens may have altered immune responses. The ability to maintain mice as specific pathogen-free depends upon the containment level of the animal facility and the housing conditions of the mice.
7. There are advantages to using female mice for intravenous infection. Male mice tend to fight and bite each other's tails, with scars making i.v. injections more difficult.

8. In our experiments, we tend to use mice within a defined age group (6–8 weeks). This is of importance as older mice have been shown to be more susceptible to *C. albicans* i.v. challenge [28, 29]. If mice of different ages must be used within an experiment, it is important to ensure that the different groups of mice are age-matched.
9. Housing conditions for mice, including number of mice per cage and the cage area required per mouse, will be dictated by local regulations. Mice infected with different *C. albicans* strains should not be maintained in the same cage.
10. Mouse tail veins are considerably easier to visualize in mice that have previously been warmed under a heat lamp or in a warm box. Mice only require a few minutes of exposure under the heat lamp; however, heating in a warm box can require heating periods of up to 30 min. Local rules may determine which method can be used to heat mice. Mice being heated by either method must never be left unsupervised and should be removed from the heat source before they show signs of overheating (lying prostrate and/or gasping).
11. Mice handled in a competent manner do not require anesthesia or sedation for tail vein injection; indeed, anesthesia can lead to increased stress and suffering. However, the use of a good mouse restraining device is essential for good i.v. injections. A number of different devices can be made or purchased. These range from modified 50 mL centrifuge tubes to commercially produced plastic holders. Holders should allow the mouse to feel secure, while allowing the investigator to hold and manipulate the tail.
12. Needles come in a variety of lengths; for i.v. injection, 10–13 mm needles are the most suitable.
13. Research involving experimental animals is differentially regulated in different parts of the world. The Animal Care and Use Committee controls animal research at Institutions in the USA, while a single EU directive covers animal research in the European Union. However, there is considerable variation in legislation in different European countries and it is essential to ensure that the correct licenses and approvals are obtained prior to beginning any study.
14. The methods permitted for humane termination of mice due to illness or at sampling times may be determined by Institutional and/or Governmental regulations. Specialist training and approval may be required to prior to use of any of the termination methods.
15. The inoculum level chosen for a specific experiment is determined by the *C. albicans* isolate/strain, the fungal growth conditions used, the mouse strain, and the infection level required. In all cases, pilot experiments should be carried out to optimize the inoculum level for any given set of conditions.

A new investigator should practice preparing inocula on several occasions prior to inocula preparation for mouse infection to ensure a good correlation between the desired inoculum level and the actual inoculum as determined by viable cell count.

In our work, we use inocula levels where control mice routinely survive for approximately 7 days. For example, for *C. albicans* isolate SC5314 grown in NGY medium and used to infect female BALB/c mice (specific pathogen-free, 6–8 weeks old) an inoculum of approximately 3×10^4 CFU per g mouse body weight is required for survival times of 5–7 days [21].

16. A mouse has three visible blood vessels; one runs down the center of the tail, with two more visible lateral tail veins running down either side of the tail (approximately 90° from the center line). These lateral tail veins should be used for i.v. infection. Often one vein appears to be more visible than the other due to lighting conditions, but either vein can be used as this does not affect infection development [14].
17. All air bubbles must be removed from syringes prior to dispensing fungal cells into the mouse bloodstream. Holding the syringe in an upright position, flick the syringe, and depress the plunger until liquid erupts from the needle. Air bubbles introduced into the bloodstream leads to immediate signs of distress (immobility and rapid heartbeat) and the mouse should be terminated immediately.

Acknowledgments

Research in the laboratory of DMM is supported by grants from the Wellcome Trust (089930), EC (STRIFE) and National Centre for the Replacement, Reduction and Refinement of Animals in Research (NC3Rs).

References

1. Kontoyiannis DP, Marr KA, Park BJ et al (2010) Prospective surveillance for invasive fungal infections in hematopoietic stem cell transplant recipients, 2001–2006: overview of the transplant-associated infection surveillance network (TRANSNET) database. Clin Infect Dis 50:1091–1100
2. Pappas PG, Alexander BD, Andes DR et al (2010) Invasive fungal infections among organ transplant recipients: results of the transplant-associated infection surveillance network (TRANSNET). Clin Infect Dis 50:1101–1111
3. Holley A, Dulhunty J, Blot S, Lipman J, Lobo S, Dancer C, Rello J, Dimopoulos G (2009) Temporal trends, risk factors and outcomes in *albicans* and non-*albicans* candidaemia: an international epidemiological study in four multidisciplinary intensive care units. Int J Antimicrob Agents 33:554.e1–554.e7
4. Horn DL, Neofytos D, Anaissie EJ, Fishman JA, Steinbach WJ, Olyaei AJ, Marr KA, Pfaller MA, Chang CH, Webster KM (2009) Epidemiology and outcomes of candidemia in 2019 patients: data from the prospective antifungal therapy alliance registry. Clin Infect Dis 48:1695–1703
5. MacCallum DM (2010) *Candida* infections and modelling disease. In: Ashbee HR, Bignell

E (eds) Pathogenic yeasts, the yeast handbook. Springer, New York, pp 41–67

6. Graf K, Khani SM, Ott E, Mattner F, Gastmeier P, Sohr D, Ziesing S, Chaberny IF (2011) Five-years surveillance of invasive aspergillosis in a university hospital. BMC Infect Dis 11:163
7. Latge JP (1999) *Aspergillus fumigatus* and aspergillosis. Clin Microbiol Rev 12:310–350
8. Chamilos G, Luna M, Lewis RE, Bodey GP, Chemaly R, Tarrand JJ, Safdar A, Raad II, Kontoyiannis DP (2006) Invasive fungal infections in patients with hematologic malignancies in a tertiary care cancer center: an autopsy study over a 15-year period (1989–2003). Haematologica 91:986–989
9. Anane S, Khalfallah F (2007) Biological diagnosis of systemic candidiasis: difficulties and future prospects. Pathol Biol 55:262–272
10. Cuenca-Estrella M, Bassetti M, Lass-Florl C, Racil Z, Richardson M, Rogers TR (2011) Detection and investigation of invasive mould disease. J Antimicrob Chemother 66(Suppl 1): i15–i24
11. Morace G, Borghi E (2010) Fungal infections in ICU patients: epidemiology and the role of diagnostics. Minerva Anestesiol 76:950–956
12. MacCallum DM (2012) Mouse intravenous challenge models and applications. Meth Mol Biol 845:499–509
13. Szabo EK, MacCallum DM (2011) The contribution of mouse models to our understanding of systemic candidiasis. FEMS Microbiol Lett 320:1–8
14. MacCallum DM, Odds FC (2005) Temporal events in the intravenous challenge model for experimental *Candida albicans* infections in female mice. Mycoses 48:151–161
15. Louria DB, Brayton RG, Finkel G (1963) Studies on the pathogenesis of experimental *Candida albicans* infections in mice. Sabouraudia 2:271–283
16. Lionakis MS, Lim JK, Lee CC, Murphy PM (2011) Organ-specific innate immune responses in a mouse model of invasive candidiasis. J Innate Immun 3:180–199
17. Spellberg B, Johnston D, Phan QT, Edwards JE Jr, French SW, Ibrahim AS, Filler SG (2003) Parenchymal organ, and not splenic, immunity correlates with host survival during disseminated candidiasis. Infect Immun 71: 5756–5764
18. MacCallum DM (2009) Massive induction of innate immune response to *Candida albicans* in the kidney in a murine intravenous challenge model. FEMS Yeast Res 9:1111–1122
19. Spellberg B, Ibrahim AS, Edwards JE Jr, Filler SG (2005) Mice with disseminated candidiasis die of progressive sepsis. J Infect Dis 192: 336–343
20. MacCallum DM, Castillo L, Brown AJP, Gow NAR, Odds FC (2009) Early-expressed chemokines predict kidney immunopathology in experimental disseminated *Candida albicans* infections. PLoS One 4:e6420
21. MacCallum DM, Castillo L, Nather K, Munro CA, Brown AJ, Gow NA, Odds FC (2009) Property differences among the four major *Candida albicans* strain clades. Eukaryot Cell 8:373–387
22. Asmundsdottir LR, Erlendsdottir H, Agnarsson BA, Gottfredsson M (2009) The importance of strain variation in virulence of *Candida dubliniensis* and *Candida albicans*: results of a blinded histopathological study of invasive candidiasis. Clin Microbiol Infect 15:576–585
23. Selmecki A, Bergmann S, Berman J (2005) Comparative genome hybridization reveals widespread aneuploidy in *Candida albicans* laboratory strains. Mol Microbiol 55:1553–1565
24. Odds FC, Van Nuffel L, Gow NA (2000) Survival in experimental *Candida albicans* infections depends on inoculum growth conditions as well as animal host. Microbiology 146:1881–1889
25. Hector RF, Domer JE, Carrow EW (1982) Immune responses to *Candida albicans* in genetically distinct mice. Infect Immun 38:1020–1028
26. Marquis G, Montplaisir S, Pelletier M, Mousseau S, Auger P (1986) Strain-dependent differences in susceptibility of mice to experimental candidosis. J Infect Dis 154:906–909
27. Ashman RB, Fulurija A, Papadimitriou JM (1996) Strain-dependent differences in host response to *Candida albicans* infection in mice are related to organ susceptibility and infectious load. Infect Immun 64:1866–1869
28. Murciano C, Yanez A, O'Connor JE, Gozalbo D, Gil ML (2008) Influence of aging on murine neutrophil and macrophage function against *Candida albicans*. FEMS Immunol Med Microbiol 53:214–221
29. Ashman RB, Papadimitriou JM, Fulurija A (1999) Acute susceptibility of aged mice to infection with *Candida albicans*. J Med Microbiol 48:1095–1102

Chapter 18

Endotoxin-Induced Uveitis in Rodents

Umesh C.S. Yadav and Kota V. Ramana

Abstract

Uveitis is a common cause of vision loss, accounting for 10–15 % of all cases of blindness worldwide and affects individuals of all ages, genders, and races. Uveitis represents a broad range of intraocular inflammatory conditions due to complications of autoimmune diseases, bacterial infections, viral infections, and chemical and metabolic injuries. Endotoxin-induced uveitis (EIU) in rodents is an efficient experimental model to investigate the pathological mechanism and pharmacological efficacy of potential drug agents. EIU is characterized by clinically relevant classical signs of inflammation, including inflammatory exudates and cells in the anterior and vitreous chambers. EIU in small animal models such as rats, mice, and rabbits is a short-lived uveal inflammation that can be developed subsequent to administration of bacterial endotoxin, such as lipopolysaccharide. Here, we present a reproducible, reliable, and simplified protocol to induce EIU in mice. This method could be used with similar efficacy for EIU induction in other small animals as well.

Key words Endotoxin-induced uveitis, Mouse, Eyes, LPS, Inflammation

1 Introduction

Uveitis was historically considered to be a single disease entity. However, as knowledge of the disease process grew with increased sophistication of immunological and microbiological testing, and biochemical and molecular techniques, it became evident that uveitis actually involves a multitude of diseases [1, 2]. Uveitis is a common cause of vision loss, accounting for 10–15 % of all cases of blindness worldwide and affects individuals of all ages, genders, and races [3, 4]. In the USA, uveitis is reportedly responsible for an estimated 30,000 new cases of legal blindness annually, and is on the rise [5]. Although prevalence studies have shown that anterior uveitis is by far the most common type, there are also posterior forms of intraocular inflammation [6]. The complications of autoimmune diseases, bacterial infections, viral infections, and chemical and metabolic injuries are associated with a variety of molecular and biochemical events that lead to ocular inflammation, particularly uveitis [7]. Furthermore, many chronic inflammatory diseases

Irving C. Allen (ed.), *Mouse Models of Innate Immunity: Methods and Protocols*, Methods in Molecular Biology, vol. 1031, DOI 10.1007/978-1-62703-481-4_18, © Springer Science+Business Media, LLC 2013

are associated with an elevated risk of uveitis, including juvenile arthritis, systemic lupus erythematosus, polyarteritis nodosa, relapsing polychondritis, Wegener's granulomatosis, Behcet's disease, and ankylosing spondylitis [8].

While it is not clear how uveitis is initiated during chronic inflammation, accumulating evidence strongly supports the association between inflammation and uveitis. Furthermore, the breakdown of the blood–aqueous barrier in uveitis involves cellular infiltration, an increase in protein permeability, upregulation of cytokines, such as TNF-α and IL-6, chemokines such as MCP-1 and MIP-1, adhesion molecules, such as ICAM-1, E-Selectins, and P-Selectins in the aqueous humor (AqH) and uveal regions. Thus, exposure of ocular tissues near the blood-aqueous barrier to inflammatory cytokines and chemokines can trigger various autocrine/paracrine effects that can eventually cause cytotoxicity, leading to blindness.

Until 1980, there were no appropriate animal models to study such a varied pathophysiology of uveitis in humans. Rosenbaum et al. for the first time reported that a systemic immunization with endotoxin produced bilateral acute anterior uveitis in rats [6]. Bacterial lipopolysaccharide (LPS) is a component of the outer envelope of all Gram-negative bacteria and a highly pro-inflammatory endotoxin. It is released from the surface of replicating Gram-negative bacteria into the circulation, where it is recognized by a variety of circulating cell types. This recognition triggers the gene induction of pro-inflammatory cytokines, such as TNF-α, IL-1, and the biosynthesis of prostaglandins (including PGE2) [6]. These and other cytokines act in an autocrine or paracrine manner and induce the breakdown of the blood–ocular barrier. This results in the infiltration of leukocytes into ocular tissues where they induce chronic inflammatory processes. The inflammation peaks 24 h after the LPS injection [6]. Although EIU was originally used as a model of anterior uveitis, increasing evidence shows that it also involves inflammation in the posterior segment of the eye, with recruitment of leukocytes that adhere to the retinal vasculature and infiltrate the vitreous cavity [9].

The discovery that the rodent EIU model mimics many of the immunopathogenic mechanisms associated with human uveitis is of great importance in developing novel therapeutic approaches [8, 10]. A number of endotoxin-induced uveitis protocols are utilized in mouse models, which include intraocular, tail vein, footpad, and subcutaneous injections of LPS. However, the varied methods and routes generate inconsistency in the disease severity, which makes the identification of disease mechanisms unreliable and the assessment of pharmacological agents questionable. Further, some routes of administration may become painful to the animals and require additional approval from appropriate regulatory agencies. Here, we describe a well-established model of LPS-induced uveitis using a simple subcutaneous injection of LPS in the thighs. The ability to induce EIU within hours using LPS in various gene-manipulated mice, including transgenic and knockout mouse strains, makes the EIU model suitable for the study of basic mechanisms and clinically relevant interventions. Thus, this model is not only simple for the induction of disease but also significantly less painful to the animals as compared to previously established footpad injection models.

2 Materials

2.1 Chemicals and Supplies for the Induction and Assessment of EIU

1. Prepare fresh solutions and reagents using molecular grade water or phosphate buffered saline (PBS) as required/indicated. Bring the solutions to room temperature before injecting into the animals. The chemicals and consumables should be disposed as per the appropriate disposal regulations for biohazard materials.
2. LPS from *Escherichia coli* (Strain 0111:B4).
3. Prepare fresh 1 mg/mL of LPS in Phosphate-buffered saline (PBS) without calcium and magnesium. Vortex at full speed on a bench top vertex for 3–5 min. Store at 4 °C or on ice.
4. 1 mL insulin syringe with permanently attached needle (27 G × 1/2 in).
5. Prepare a Glutalardehyde (1 %) and paraformaldehyde (4 %) mixture in PBS and store at room temperature. Aliquot 20 mL of the fixative per 3–4 eyes in flat bottom glass vials.
6. 1.5 mL Eppendorf tubes.
7. 15 and 50 mL centrifuge tubes.
8. Dissection instruments: microdissection scissors; forceps; and scalpel.

2.2 Animals

1. Six to eight weeks-old, 25–30 g C57Bl/6 mice (*see* **Notes 1** and **2**).
2. House the animals in a 12 h day night cycle with standard chow and water ad libitum.
3. Acclimate the mice at least 3–4 days prior to experiments.

3 Methods

3.1 Induction of Endotoxin-Induced Uveitis

1. Prepare fresh LPS and keep on ice.
2. Prepare a cotton ball or a wipe with 70 % alcohol for disinfection and to smoothen out the body hairs (alternatively mice can be shaved before applying the alcohol on both the thighs to make the skin accessible).
3. Assemble a syringe with a 27 G × 1/2″ needle and fill with 100 μL of LPS solution (containing 100 μg of LPS/mouse) (*see* **Notes 3** and **4**). Remove any air bubbles and place the syringe in a sterile tray.

4. To restrain the mouse, remove the animal from the cage and have an assistant hold the animal by its scruff parallel to the table. Stabilize the mouse on the bench (*see* **Note 5**).
5. Hold the animal's hind leg with the nondominant hand, presenting the side surface for injection.
6. Swab the right thigh with a 70 % alcohol drenched cotton ball so that the hairs are smoothened and the skin is visible.
7. Hold the syringe in the dominant hand and place the needle on the thigh at a 5–10° angle.
8. Slide the needle in the forward direction penetrating the skin. Advance the needle further into skin until the entire bevel is inside the skin. Take special care to avoid entering the muscle.
9. At this point, inject 50 μL of the LPS solution with minimal movement (*see* **Note 6**).
10. If the subcutaneous injection is performed properly, a bubble or a slight raised area should be observed under the skin at the injection site. If a bubble is not formed, the LPS has either dispersed rapidly or was injected into the muscle.
11. Withdraw the needle and securely place it back into the syringe tray.
12. Repeat the procedure for the other leg.
13. After injecting in both of the thighs, return the animal to the cage and mark the cage card.
14. As an alternative procedure, the animals can be sedated with isoflurane immediately prior to the subcutaneous LPS injection.
15. If performing therapeutic agent studies, the animals can be randomly segregated into different experimental groups. The therapeutic agent can be administered either prior to the LPS injection or 1–2 h post LPS injection.
16. Return all the animals to their respective cages and leave the animals with their chow and drinking water.
17. Examine the eyes for pathological signs at different time intervals as needed.

3.2 Assessment of Uveitis: Pathological Score

1. The disease progression can be assessed in the animals starting 3 h post LPS injection and continued at a desired time interval until 24 h. The disease progression reaches its peak at 24 h and begins to resolve. Additional time points typically include 48 h and during disease resolution.
2. For clinical assessment, anesthetize the animals using appropriate doses of pentobarbital (30–60 mg/kg body weight) or any other agent as recommend by your institute's veterinarian.
3. Bring one animal under the surgical microscope, open the eye lid and examine it for any of the following signs of disease: signs of

cellular infiltration in the anterior chamber; vessel dilation; fibrinoid exudates; and flair and turbidity due to protein exudation.

4. After examination, the pathological scores are assigned to each eye based on the following grading scale: 0, no inflammatory reaction; 1, discrete inflammatory reaction; 2, moderate dilation of the iris and conjunctiva vessels; 3, intense iridial hyperemia, with flare in the anterior chamber; and 4, same signs as in grade 3 with the addition of fibrinoid exudation in the papillary area and intense flare in the anterior chamber.
5. The animals may be returned to their cages to revive, or euthanized appropriately for histopathological assessments.

3.3 Extraction of Aqueous Humor

1. Aqueous humor (AqH) is an important source of assessing inflammatory changes such as cellular infiltration, protein exudation, release of cytokines and chemokines in the anterior chamber. However, extraction of AqH is easier in rats and rabbits as compared to mice due to the size of the eye balls (*see* **Note 7**).
2. To extract the AqH from mouse eyes, place the euthanized animals under the surgical microscope.
3. Insert 29 G needle with a syringe through the corner of conjunctiva and enter the anterior chamber by piercing the cornea and simultaneously withdrawing the plunger to extract the AqH.
4. Because of positive pressure AqH has a tendency to ooze out as soon as the cornea is punctured; therefore, one should draw the plunger while entering the eye to minimize the loss of AqH. Practice is needed to perform this procedure.
5. Transfer the AqH (4–8 μL/mice) in an eppendorf tube and store on ice.
6. Dilute appropriately and use for assessments of protein and cellular infiltrates in the AqH.
7. Store the AqH at −80 °C for the determination of cytokines and chemokines.

3.4 Enucleating of Eyes

1. The eyes can be enucleated using a fine surgical scissor and forceps.
2. Make a fine incision around the conjunctiva without cutting any blood vessels.
3. In order to cut the optic nerve and set the eye ball free, probe deep into the ocular cavity with a scissor. Cut the optic nerve and take out the eye ball.
4. Clean the attached muscles and hairs (if any) and immediately immerse the eye ball in the fixative solution aliquoted in a glass vial.
5. Incubate the vials at room temperature for 24 h.
6. Transfer the eyes to 70 % alcohol (histopathological grade) and keep at room temperature for 24 h.

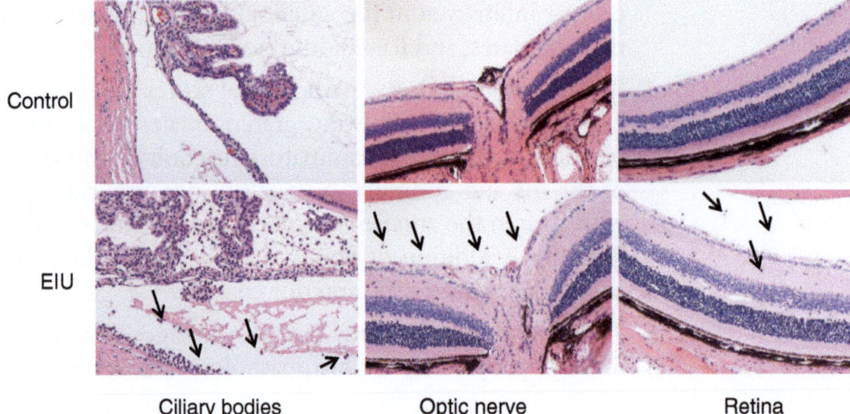

Fig. 1 Histopathological evaluation of EIU in mice. Twenty-four hours after LPS injection in mice, the eye sections were stained with H&E. *Arrows* show the infiltration of inflammatory cells (leukocytes) in the ciliary bodies, optic nerve, and retinal regions of the mouse eyes

7. Transfer the eye balls to 90 % alcohol and process them for paraffin embedding and sectioning (5 μM) using standard histological procedures.
8. Stain the eye sections with Hematoxylin and Eosin (H&E) using a standard protocol.
9. Examine the eye sections under a bright field microscope for histopathological symptoms and grade.

3.5 Histopathological Grading

1. For histopathological evaluation, H&E stained eye sections can be observed under a light microscope.
2. The Iris–ciliary body complex, anterior chamber, posterior chamber, vitreous, and retina may be observed for the inflammatory cell infiltration, blood vessel dilation, and any damage in the ocular tissues (Fig. 1) (*see* **Note 8**).
3. The histological grading of the eye section can be performed on the basis of cellular infiltrates in the anterior chamber (*see* **Note 9**).

4 Notes

1. This protocol can be adapted for a variety of animals, including mouse, rabbit, guinea pig, or rat.
2. The standard deviation and severity of the disease can vary greatly depending on the genetic background of the animal used. For example, we have shown that C57Bl6 mice develop the best EIU [11].
3. The dose of LPS should be standardized for each experiment. We observed that a subcutaneous dose of 50 μg/mouse of

LPS per thigh is enough to induce effective EIU symptoms. The disease can also be induced by footpad injection, but there are restrictions to this method as outlined by The Association for Research in Vision and Ophthalmology (ARVO) and the National Institutes of Health (NIH) policy on animal use in research [11].

4. The dose of the LPS also depends on the route of administration. Systemic injection of LPS provides a more clinically relevant disease condition.
5. Every precaution should be taken in animal handling and disposal of animal waste as outlined by the Institutional Ethics committee and animal protocol approval.
6. LPS is biohazardous and proper protection equipment should be worn during the procedures described in this protocol.
7. Extraction of AqH in rats is easier compared to mice. The volume of AqH recovered from a rat is around 10–15 μL. However, it is possible to extract AqH from mice, but it is more tedious and requires better skills. As an alternative or complementary assessment, mouse eye histopathology sections can be used to examine inflammatory changes.
8. Shen et al. pointed out the biphasic nature of endotoxin-induced uveitis in mice, which may be a better experimental model given the recurrent nature of human uveitis [12].
9. In addition to EIU, experimental autoimmune uveitis (EAU) is another animal model of inflammatory eye disease that mimics endogenous posterior uveoretinitis and is thought to have an autoimmune origin [13]. EAU is a well-characterized, robust, and reproducible model. However, the disease peaks in 2–3 weeks depending on the animal species. Immunization of animals at distant sites with retinal antigens and appropriate adjuvant results in a disease with many of the clinical and histopathological features associated with the human disease.

Acknowledgments

This work in the author's lab was supported by National Institutes of Health (NIH) Grant EY015891 to K.V.R.

References

1. de Smet MD, Taylor SR, Bodaghi B et al (2011) Understanding uveitis: the impact of research on visual outcomes. Prog Retin Eye Res 30:452–470
2. Rathinam SR, Namperumalsamy P (2007) Global variation and pattern changes in epidemiology of uveitis. Indian J Ophthalmol 55:173–183
3. Nussenblatt RB (1990) The natural history of uveitis. Int Ophthalmol 14:303–308
4. Read R (2006) Uveitis: advances in understanding of pathogenesis. CurrRheumatol Rep 8:260–266
5. Gritz DC, Wong IG (2004) Incidence and prevalence of uveitis in Northern California;

the Northern California epidemiology of uveitis study. Ophthalmology 111:491–500

6. Rosenbaum JT, McDevitt HO, Guss RB et al (1980) Endotoxin induced uveitis in rats as a model for human disease. Nature 286:611–613
7. Chatzistefanou K, Markomichelakis NN, Christen W et al (1998) Characteristics of uveitis presenting for the first time in the elderly. Ophthalmology 105:347–352
8. Yadav UC, Kalariya NM, Ramana KV (2011) Emerging role of antioxidants in the protection of uveitis complications. Curr Med Chem 18:931–942
9. Altan-Yaycioglu R, Akova YA, Akca S et al (2006) Inflammation of the posterior uvea: findings on fundus fluorescein and indocyanine green angiography. Ocul Immunol Inflamm 14:171–179
10. Yadav UC, Srivastava SK, Ramana KV (2007) Aldose reductase inhibition prevents endotoxin-induced uveitis in rats. Invest Ophthalmol Vis Sci 48:4634–4642
11. Kamala T (2007) Hock immunization: a humane alternative to mouse footpad injections. J Immunol Methods 328:204–214
12. Shen DF, Chang MA, Matteson DM, Buggage R, Kozhich AT, Chan CC (2000) Biphasic ocular inflammatory response to endotoxin-induced uveitis in the mouse. Arch Ophthalmol 118:521–527
13. Yadav UC, Shoeb M, Srivastava SK, Ramana KV (2011) Aldose reductase deficiency protects from autoimmune- and endotoxin-induced uveitis in mice. Invest Ophthalmol Vis Sci 52:8076–8085

Chapter 19

Bacteria-Mediated Acute Lung Inflammation

Irving C. Allen

Abstract

Mouse models of acute lung inflammation are critical for understanding the role of the innate immune response to pathogen associated molecular patterns, bacteria, and sepsis in humans. Bacterial infections in the lung elicit a range of immune reactions, depending on the pathogen, the level of exposure and the effectiveness of the host response. In general, mice have proven to be an acceptable surrogate model organism for studying specific aspects of human lung pathogenesis, including localized and systemic inflammation, necrotizing pneumonia, bacteriemia, and survival. Here, we describe a highly versatile model utilizing the gram-negative bacterium *Klebsiella pneumoniae*. Following a single challenge with this bacterium, mice develop a robust Th1 mediated immune response and clinically relevant disease progression. While these protocols have been optimized for *K. pneumoniae*, they can be applied to any gram-positive or gram-negative organism of interest.

Key words *Klebisella pneumoniae*, Necrosis, Lung inflammation, Pneumonia, Pulmonary infection, Macrophage, Neutrophil, Th1, Gram-negative bacteria

1 Introduction

Acute respiratory diseases such as pathogen mediated infections and pneumonia represent a significant public health burden, which is expected to increase in the coming decades. Elucidating the underlying mechanisms associated with the host innate immune response to the agents associated with these diseases will facilitate the development of innovative prevention strategies and novel therapeutic agents targeting these infections. One pathogen of specific relevance to acute respiratory disease is *Klebsiella pneumoniae*. *K. pneumoniae* is a common gram-negative bacterium and is a normal component of the mouth, skin and intestinal microbiome. The bacteria are nonmotile, non-flagellated, and rod-shaped. *K. pneumoniae* is routinely encountered by clinicians and is a leading cause of respiratory infections [1]. It has been estimated that up to 23 % of all nosocomial infections are associated with *K. pneumoniae* and infection with this bacterium is of

Irving C. Allen (ed.), *Mouse Models of Innate Immunity: Methods and Protocols*, Methods in Molecular Biology, vol. 1031, DOI 10.1007/978-1-62703-481-4_19, © Springer Science+Business Media, LLC 2013

particular concern as it carries a mortality rate of up 50 % in the elderly or immunocompromised individuals [2]. Over the last decade, clinicians have reported a growing prevalence of antibiotic resistant strains of this species [3, 4]. In humans, pathogenic *K. pneumoniae* lung infections are capable of inducing severe bacterial pneumonia, which often progresses to bacteremia and sepsis [5]. The acute lung infection typically results in extensive tissue injury associated with excessive inflammation, hemorrhage and necrotic damage. These latter symptoms result in the characteristic thick, blood-laced mucus that is often described as "currant jelly" sputum. Significant progress has been made in characterizing the innate immune mechanisms associated with the diverse host responses elicited by *K. pneumoniae* [6–9].

Here, we describe a highly flexible model of acute lung inflammation that is based on *Klebsiella pneumoniae* infection. In our hands, this model successfully recapitulates many physiologically relevant aspects of gram-negative bacterial infection and acute necrotizing pneumonia in humans. The protocols presented here are designed to maximize the data generated from individual mice and minimize the number of animals required to complete studies. In addition, we also present alternative protocols to evaluate specific aspects of acute lung inflammation that are often overlooked by typical studies. This model is easily adaptable to evaluate other gram-negative and gram-positive bacterial infections in the lungs, as well as other viral, fungal, or damage associated airway inflammation models.

2 Materials

2.1 Mice

1. Adult mice, 6–12 weeks old (*see* **Note 1**) that have been bred and housed under specific pathogen free conditions (*see* **Note 2**).
2. Mice should be acclimated to the housing facility for at least 5 days prior to the beginning of the experiment.

2.2 Reagents and Solutions

1. *Klebsiella pneumoniae*, serotype 2 (American Type Culture Collection (ATCC), VA, USA) (*see* **Note 3**).
2. Nutrient Agar (Becton, Dickinson and Company, NJ, USA).
3. Nutrient Broth (Becton, Dickinson and Company, NJ, USA).
4. Deionized water.
5. Gentamicin.
6. 1× Hank's Buffered Saline Solution (HBSS).
7. 10× Phosphate Buffered Saline (PBS).
8. Sterile Water.
9. Isoflurane (*see* **Note 4**).

10. 10× Buffered Formalin.
11. Trypan Blue.
12. Formamide.
13. Diff-Quick Staining Kit.
14. Permount.
15. ELISA Kits for IL-1β, IL-6, and TNFα.
16. Liquid Nitrogen.
17. Standard reagents for RNA extraction, cDNA amplification, and real-time PCR analysis.
18. Standard reagents for protein extraction and Western blot analysis.

2.3 Materials and Equipment for Innoculation

1. 37 °C incubator for culturing bacteria, which should be separate and distinct from any utilized for routine tissue culture.
2. Platform shaker.
3. 50 ml flask.
4. UV/Vis spectrophotometer with cuvettes.
5. Glass beads or plate spreader for plating bacteria.
6. Chamber for drop method anesthesia (i.e., 500 ml beaker with lid).
7. p200 pipette.
8. Forceps.
9. Rodent intubation stand.

2.4 Materials and Equipment for Post-innoculation Monitoring

1. Small animal rectal thermometer.
2. Digital scale.

2.5 Materials and Equipment for Animal Harvest

1. 1 ml Syringe (with 27 gage needle).
2. 1.5 ml microcentrifuge tubes.
3. Microcentrifuge.
4. p1000 pipette.
5. 10 ml Syringe (with 27 gage needle).
6. Three 1 ml Syringes (without needles).
7. 15 ml conical tubes.
8. Tracheal Cannula (*see* **Note 5**) (Harvard Apparatus, MA, USA).
9. 4-0, Silk Surgical Suture.
10. Refrigerated benchtop centrifuge (with rotor to accommodate 15 ml conical tubes).

11. Hemacytometer.
12. Microscope (10× and 20× objectives).
13. Cytospin.
14. Microscope Slides.
15. Coverslips.
16. Coplin Jars.
17. 10 ml syringe with a 6 in. piece of medical tubing fitted at the hub.
18. 20 ml disposable glass scintillation vials with lids.
19. Tissue homogenizer.
20. 5 ml syringe (without needle).
21. Portable Liquid Nitrogen container or bucket.
22. Fine tipped indelible marker.
23. 2 ml screw-cap cryo tubes.
24. Mouse necropsy tools: 1 pair of large blunt scissors, 1 pair of straight forceps, 1 pair of blunt 90° angled forceps, 1 pair of sharp 90° angled scissors, 1 pair of slightly curved blunt scissors.

3 Methods

3.1 Prepare K. pneumoniae and Culture Bacteria in Nutrient Broth

1. With a sterilized inoculating loop, streak a nutrient agar plate to isolate single colonies from the bacteria stock. Incubate the plate at 37 °C overnight.
2. Select a single colony from the plate using a sterilized pipette tip or inoculating loop and inoculate 20 ml of nutrient broth in a small flask. Seal the remaining plate with paraffin and store at 4 °C for up to 1 week.
3. *K. pneumoniae* can be cultured in a variety of broths and agars. However, we recommend using the suggested reagents from the bacteria stock supplier, in this case ATCC. Bacteria growth is rapid at 37 °C and oxygenation of the cultures is recommended though shaking during incubation. Under these conditions, we have found that *K. pneumoniae* divide in broth culture approximately every 20–30 min.
4. Monitor and quantify bacteria growth during early log-phase cultures using light absorbance at A_{600}. In our experience, 1 OD600 = 3×10^8 bacteria/ml. However, this was determined through empirical testing and should be evaluated prior to the start of these experiments.
5. Dilute the bacteria to deliver 7.4×10^4 CFUs of *K. pneumoniae* in 50 μl of 1× PBS/mouse, as previously described [9]. Store on ice until ready for use.

3.2 K. pneumoniae Lung Innoculation Using i.t. Administration (See Note 6)

1. Baseline body weight and body temperature should be recorded immediately prior to *K. pneumoniae* instillation.
2. Withdraw the 50 μl bacteria dose from the inoculum prepared above.
3. Anesthetize a mouse using drop method isoflurane in the 500 ml beaker with glass cover (*see* **Note 7**).
4. Mice should be placed on the intubation stand and gently secured by their incisors as directed by the stand's manufacturer.
5. Gently pull the mouse's tongue straight out using forceps. This effectively repositions the epiglottis and allows access to the trachea.
6. While still holding the tongue in position, dispense the 50 μl bacteria dose in the back of the mouth and throat. Place fingers over the mouse's nose. The mouse will eventually aspirate the bacteria inoculum, which typically results in a characteristic crackle sound that is audible shortly after inspiration.
7. Once the mouse has aspirated the bacteria dose, gently remove the animal from the intubation rack and place it back in a clean cage for recovery.
8. Immediately following i.t. administration, a subset of animals should be euthanized and the lungs harvested to evaluate bacteria CFUs, as described below, to determine the actual dose given to each animal.
9. Survival, body weight and body temperature are effective surrogate markers of disease progression [9]. Within the first 4–6 h, animals will demonstrate a significant decrease in body temperature that will peak within the first 24 h after challenge. Body temperature will gradually recover within 48 h as the animals begin to clear the bacteria. Concurrent with temperature decreases, body weight will also begin to decline within the first 24 h and peak at approximately 48 h following bacteria challenge. Thus, within the first 72 h, mice should be monitored up to three times per day and moribund animals should be sacrificed following appropriate institutional specific guidelines.

3.3 Tissue Collection to Evaluate the Host Innate Immune Response

1. 48–72 h following the bacteria exposure, euthanize the mice following appropriate institutional guidelines (*see* **Note 8**). This time range represents the typical peak in the host innate immune response to the bacteria. However, this timing should be modified based on the experimental goals of each individual study.
2. For systemic assessments of circulating cytokines, whole blood should be collected utilizing cardiac puncture immediately following euthanasia (*see* **Note 9**). The whole blood should be

allowed to coagulate at room temperature for at least 30 min prior to serum isolation.

3. Perfuse the animals using 1× HBSS. Carefully open the peritoneal cavity and cut the portal vein leading to the kidney (either side). This will allow the remaining blood to drain from the animal during the perfusion. Without opening the chest, carefully move the liver to expose the diaphragm. The lungs and heart should be visible behind the translucent diaphragm. Carefully clip the diaphragm at the point of contact with the sternum, making a small nick to access the chest. Once the nick is generated, the lungs and tissues should resend into the chest cavity. The bottom of the heart should now be visible. Using a 10 ml syringe with 27 gage needle attached, slowly and carefully inject the heart. Gently inject 1–3 ml of HBSS. The lungs should begin to change color from red to pinkish/white and the liquid flowing from the excised kidney should change from red to clear. Use caution when injecting HBSS into the heart. If too much pressure is applied to the syringe, saline can be forced into the airways and compromise additional data collection.
4. Once the animal has been perfused, the chest cavity can be exposed. Using a pair of blunt scissors, carefully open the chest cavity and remove each side of the rib cage as completely as possible and without damaging the lungs. Next, carefully remove the collar bones, taking care to not damage the underling trachea. Using blunt tipped forceps, separate the salivary glands and remove the thin layer of muscle that lies overtop of the trachea in the mouse's neck. The trachea should now be exposed from the lungs to the larynx.
5. Using the 90° angled sharp scissors, make a small incision in the trachea 1–3 tracheal rings below the larynx. The incision should be just large enough to insert and secure the tracheal cannula. Do not sever the trachea as this will cause the trachea to retract into the chest cavity. Insert the tracheal cannula into the incision. Brace the trachea with the straight blunt forceps. Using the 90° angled blunt forceps, thread the suture directly under the trachea and securely tie the cannula into place.
6. Collect the BALF. Fill a 50 ml conical tube with 1× HBSS. Fill three 1 ml syringes (without needles) with 1 ml of HBSS. Ensure that no bubbles are present in the syringe, and that the HBSS is flush with the end of the syringe. Gently attach the hub of the syringe to the tracheal cannula and slowly inject 900 μl of HBSS into the mouse lungs in one continuous motion. The lungs should visibly inflate with no obvious leaks. Immediately withdraw the fluid, also in one slow and continuous motion. Deposit the BALF into a 15 ml conical tube on ice. Repeat this process with the other two syringes. However, subsequent lavages should utilize the full 1 ml of HBSS per

lavage. Record the final volume of BALF collected for each animal. The final volume should be approximately 3 ml total. Keep the BALF on ice until ready for further evaluation.

7. Inflate the lungs and fix for histopathology. Fill the 10 ml syringe with attached tubing with 10 % buffered formalin. Brace the trachea with the straight blunt forceps. Using the 90° angled blunt forceps, thread a second suture directly under the trachea and below the end of the cannula. Loop the suture in a half tightened knot. Do not completely tighten the knot. Insert the tube from the 10 ml syringe into the cannula hub. Gently inflate the lungs with approximately 1 ml of 10 % buffered formalin. Do not overinflate the lungs as this will result in distortions in the lung histopathology. Once the lungs are inflated, secure the knot on the half tied suture. Remove the syringe, tubing and cannula from the trachea. Grasp the excess suture thread with the forceps and gently lift the trachea. Using the curved blunt scissors, slowly severe the trachea while lifting the inflated lungs out of the chest cavity. Carefully excise the lungs (with the heart still attached) without cutting them. Gently remove the inflated lungs from the mouse. Place the inflated lungs in a 20 ml disposable glass scintillation vial containing approximately 10 ml of 10 % buffered formalin. Place a lid on the vial and label with an indelible pen.
8. Properly dispose of the remaining mouse carcass.

3.4 Tissue Collection to Evaluate Bacteria Clearance and Gene Expression Profiling

1. In addition to evaluating the host innate immune response, it is also desirable to evaluate bacteria growth and clearance in the lung, as well as, bacterial translocation to distal tissues including the liver and spleen [10]. To evaluate these parameters, subsets of animals from each experimental and control group should be harvested for tissue extraction and homogenization.
2. Euthanize the mice, collect the whole blood via heart stick and perfuse the mice as described in Protocol 3.3, **steps 1–3**. Once the animal has been perfused, the chest cavity can be exposed. Using a pair of blunt scissors, open the chest cavity and remove each side of the rib cage as completely as possible. Remove the heart and carefully remove each lung lobe individually, taking care to ensure that no lymph nodes or portions of the thymus are included. Place the lung lobes in labeled tubes on ice until ready to homogenize. In our experience, 5 ml round bottom snap cap tubes work well for this procedure.
3. Inside of a BSL2 rated biological safety cabinet, add 1 ml of 1× sterile PBS to each lung sample and completely homogenize the lungs using a tissue homogenizer. Determine lung CFUs by generating serial dilutions from the lung homogenates and plating on nutrient agar [9, 10] (*see* **Note 10**).

4. In addition to lung CFUs, the liver and spleen should also be harvested, homogenized and plated as described above to determine bacteria dissemination.
5. Following homogenization and plating, the remaining homogenates can be separated into two additional aliquots and centrifuged at 200×*g* in a microcentrifuge. Remove the supernatants and store the pellets at −80 °C until ready for RNA or protein extraction.

3.5 Sample Analysis

1. Analyze cytokine profiles in the serum. After allowing the whole blood to coagulate at room temperature for at least 30 min, spin the samples in a microcentrifuge at maximum speed (~16,200×*g*) for 5 min. Label a 1.5 ml microcentrifuge tube for serum collection with the indelible pen, one tube for each serum sample. Carefully remove the tubes containing the now separated whole blood from the centrifuge. Note the separation of the blood into two distinct phases. The serum is isolated in the top layer. Carefully remove the serum from the tube using a p1000 pipette and transfer the serum to the newly labeled microcentrifuge tube and keep on ice until ready for storage. The recovered volume of serum should be approximately equal to 20 % of the total volume of whole blood. Store the serum at −80 °C until ready for use.
2. For cytokine analysis by ELISA, the serum should be diluted 1:5–1:20 (depending on the assay). These dilutions should be empirically determined prior to running the bulk of the samples. Due to the low volume of serum collected, most sample volumes can be reduced by half for loading on the ELISA plate (i.e., most commercial ELISAs utilize 100 μl volumes of standards and samples; for serum, load 50 μl of standards and diluted samples). Common ELISAs for serum include IL-1β, IL-6, and TNFα [9, 10].
3. Analyze cytokine levels in cell free BALF. Remove 500 μl of BALF. Conduct a serial dilution of the samples for plating on nutrient agar to evaluate CFUs (*see* **Note 10**). Spin the remaining BALF in their respective 15 ml conical tubes in a refrigerated tabletop centrifuge at 200×*g* for 5 min to pellet the cells. Label two 1.5 ml microcentrifuge tubes with the indelible pen. Two tubes for each sample. Carefully remove the 15 ml tubes from the centrifuge without disturbing the cell pellet. Carefully transfer the BALF supernatant to the 1.5 ml microcentrifuge tubes and keep on ice. Store the BALF at −80 °C until ready for use.
4. For cytokine analysis by ELISA, the BALF should be used neat or diluted 1:5 (depending on the assay). These dilutions should be empirically determined prior to running the bulk of the samples. Unlike the serum, the BALF should yield ample volume for ELISA and western blot analysis. However, most

sample volumes can also be reduced by half for loading on the ELISA plate, as discussed for the serum. Common ELISAs for the BALF include IL-1β, IL-6, and TNFα [9, 10].

5. Lyse the red blood cells in the BALF using hypotonic saline (*see* **Note 11**). Following centrifugation and the complete removal of the HBSS, resuspend the cells in 900 μl of distilled water. Immediately add 100 μl of 10× PBS. Samples should be lysed one at a time. If samples contain excessive amounts of red blood cells, the cells can be pelleted in the table top centrifuge at 400 × *g* for 5 min and the red blood cell lysis protocol can be repeated.
6. Determine the total BALF cellularity in the 1 ml suspension using a hemacytometer under 10–20× magnification with Trypan Blue staining. These data can be evaluated as cells/ml [9, 10].
7. Collect cells for differential staining (*see* **Note 12**). Label standard microscope slides using a pencil or solvent resistant pen. Secure the slides into the cytospin holder and funnel. Remove 150 μl of BALF and cytospin at 100 × *g* for 5 min. The volume spun down onto the slides can be reduced if cell density is too great to evaluate cell morphology. Allow the slides to air dry overnight.
8. Differential stain the slides following the manufactures protocols. Allow the slides to air dry overnight. Coverslip the slides using permount. Evaluate the slides using a microscope equipped with a 20× and 40× objective.
9. Harvest the remaining cells for subsequent analysis, such as FACS, electron microscopy, confocal microscopy, RNA extraction for gene expression evaluation, and/or protein extraction for Western Blot. In general, these subsequent assays such as flow cytometry will be limited by the number of cells collected in the lavage. For most protocols, the cells can be concentrated by centrifugation at 200 × *g* for 5 min, the supernatant removed and samples stored at −80 °C until ready for use.
10. Prepare the lung for histopathology evaluation. After 24–48 h of formalin fixation, the whole inflated lungs should be ventrally orientated and embedded in paraffin. The resultant blocks should be cut to expose the main conducting airway. Increased scoring accuracy can be achieved by orientating the lungs in the same position and cut to the same depth. Five micron serial sections of the lungs should be cut and stained with H&E. Additional sections can be cut and prepared for in situ hybridization using standard protocols.
11. Evaluate lung histopathology using H&E scoring and evaluation. H&E staining is extremely useful in the evaluation of overall lung inflammation. The most efficient technique to evaluate

H&E staining in these types of assays is through semi-quantitative inflammation scoring of the left lung lobe. Sections of the left lobe should be cut to yield the maximum longitudinal visualization of the intrapulmonary main axial airway and evaluated by an experienced pathologist. Histopathology can then be evaluated by the following inflammatory parameters, which are scored between 0 (absent) and 3 (severe): mononuclear and polymorphonuclear cell infiltration; airway epithelial cell hyperplasia and injury; extravasation; perivascular and peribroncheolar cuffing; and the percent of the lung involved with inflammation. These parameter scores can then be averaged for a total histology score or used individually to quantify specific aspects of disease progression. Scoring should always be conducted in a double blind fashion, with reviewers blinded to both genotype and treatment. This scoring system has been previously described [9, 10].

4 Notes

1. We have successfully utilized 6–12-week-old C57Bl/6, 129SvEv, and BALB/c mice in these assays. If strain is not a limiting factor, C57Bl/6 mice are preferred due to their Th1 skewing and robust response. It is possible that some aspects of this protocol may need to be adjusted and further optimized when using mice from different genetic backgrounds.
2. All studies should be conducted in accordance with the local and institutional animal care and use guidelines and in accordance with the prevailing national regulations.
3. *K. pneumoniae* is infectious and is classified as a BSL-2 pathogen. Materials in this category present a moderate risk to laboratory personnel and should be handled under standard BSL-2 guidelines. Additional pathogen specific institutional, local, and national regulatory guidelines apply. All infectious materials should be handled under the direct supervision of competent and knowledgeable laboratory personnel. A materials transfer agreement (MTA) with ATCC is required for the use of this pathogen.
4. 2,2,2 Tribromoethanol (Avertin) is a common substitute for drop method isoflurane anesthesia in acute airway inflammation protocols. However, in our experience, the deep plain of anesthesia induced by avertin can actually reduce the effectiveness of the intratrachael administrations.
5. We recommend the use of specialized, commercially available tracheal cannulas. However, 16 gage needles can be used as substitutes. In our experience, this alternative works best when the needles are ground down to a blunt end.

6. Intratrachael administration requires extensive practice to achieve proficiency. Improper technique can result in injury to the mouse and inefficient lung delivery. However, once proficient, this technique is ideal for delivering infectious agents to the lungs and has been found to be more accurate than intranasal inoculation. In our hands, we have found that Evans Blue Dye (EBD) is an effective training tool. A 1 % solution of EBD in 1× PBS can be generated, filter sterilized and administered i.t. To quantify the efficiency of the i.t. administration, the lungs can be removed and incubated in formamide for 48 h at room temperature to extract the EBD. The absorption of Evans blue can be measured using a standard plate reader at 620 nm and deposited Evans blue can be calculated against a standard curve to quantify technique efficiency.
7. Drop method isoflurane induces a low level of anesthesia that is recommended for this procedure. We have found that light anesthesia allows for more effective i.t. instillation compared to other techniques, which often suppress breathing volumes and rates. Drop method isoflurane induces anesthesia within 30 s and will lightly anesthetize the mouse for approximately 30 s. Each individual institution will have specific guidelines regarding the use of drop method anesthesia.
8. Note that inhalation anesthetics, such as isoflurane, may result in confounding issues when studying lung physiology. Therefore, ensure that control animals are properly utilized and limit the animal's exposure to the anesthetic as much as possible.
9. The blood should be harvested by heartstick using the 1 ml syringe with a 27 gage needle attached. There are multiple approved methods of conducting the heartstick. We have found that it is most effective when performed prior to making any incisions on the animal. Immediately after removal from the CO_2 chamber, ensure proper euthanasia by toe pinch reflex and pin the mouse to a surgical board. Spray the animal with 70 % ethanol and locate the base of the sternum. Insert the needle between the last 2 ribs and slightly to the right of the center. Using a controlled and singular motion, begin withdrawing the blood from the heart. With practice, this procedure can typically recover 500–800 μl of whole blood. Transfer the blood from the syringe to a labeled 1.5 ml microcentrifuge tube. Remove the needle from the syringe prior to transferring the blood. Forcing the blood through the needle will induce cell lysis and inhibit serum collection.
10. In addition to lung CFUs generated from the lung homogenates, the BALF will also contain live bacteria and can effectively be utilized to determine bacteria load. However, BALF CFUs are often more variable then lung CFUs.

11. There are many different protocols for red blood cell lysis. The protocol described here is optimized for the subsequent basic morphology assessments by differential staining and total cell counts. However, this procedure is often considered suboptimal for higher resolution analyses, such as FACs. Red blood cell lysis via ACK lysing buffer is a viable alternative for procedures requiring less background and higher resolution.

12. Differential staining allows for morphology based identification of BALF cellularity. To ensure the optimal results, the samples should be cytospun on the same day they are collected and the staining reagents should be prepared fresh prior to each use. DiffQuick based protocols allow the differentiation of eosinophils (granules stain red) and neutrophils (granules do not stain). Monocytic cells can be easily identified, but are difficult to distinguish. Therefore, these cells should be identified as monocytes, rather than macrophages. Likewise, lymphocytes are also commonly observed in the BALF. However, it is also unlikely that typical researchers can distinguish T-cells from B-cells based on morphology alone. Thus, many investigators have modified these procedures for use with flow cytometry. The only limiting factor is the low number of total cells typically harvested from control animals. Even with flow cytometry, differential staining should be used to confirm the results.

References

1. Ko WC, Paterson DL, Sagnimeni AJ, Hansen DS, Von Gottberg A, Mohapatra S, Casellas JM, Goossens H, Mulazimoglu L, Trenholme G, Klugman KP, McCormack JG, Yu VL (2002) Community-acquired Klebsiella pneumoniae bacteremia: global differences in clinical patterns. Emerg Infect Dis 8:160–166
2. Feldman C, Ross S, Mahomed AG, Omar J, Smith C (1995) The aetiology of severe community-acquired pneumonia and its impact on initial, empiric, antimicrobial chemotherapy. Respir Med 89:187–192
3. Keynan Y, Rubinstein E (2007) The changing face of Klebsiella pneumoniae infections in the community. Int J Antimicrob Agents 30: 385–389
4. Paterson DL, Ko WC, Von Gottberg A, Mohapatra S, Casellas JM, Goossens H, Mulazimoglu L, Trenholme G, Klugman KP, Bonomo RA, Rice LB, Wagener MM, McCormack JG, Yu VL (2004) Antibiotic therapy for Klebsiella pneumoniae bacteremia: implications of production of extended-spectrum beta-lactamases. Clin Infect Dis 39:31–37
5. Sahly H, Podschun R (1997) Clinical, bacteriological, and serological aspects of Klebsiella infections and their spondylarthropathic sequelae. Clin Diagn Lab Immunol 4: 393–399
6. Ledford JG, Kovarova M, Koller BH (2007) Impaired host defense in mice lacking ONZIN. J Immunol 178:5132–5143
7. Jeyaseelan S, Young SK, Yamamoto M, Arndt PG, Akira S, Kolls JK, Worthen GS (2006) Toll/IL-1R domain-containing adaptor protein (TIRAP) is a critical mediator of antibacterial defense in the lung against Klebsiella pneumoniae but not Pseudomonas aeruginosa. J Immunol 177:538–547
8. Kostina E, Ofek I, Crouch E, Friedman R, Sirota L, Klinger G, Sahly H, Keisari Y (2005) Noncapsulated Klebsiella pneumoniae bearing mannose-containing O antigens is rapidly eradicated from mouse lung and triggers cytokine production by macrophages following opsonization with surfactant protein D. Infect Immun 73:8282–8290
9. Willingham SB, Allen IC, Bergstralh DT, Brickey WJ, Huang MT, Taxman DJ, Duncan JA, Ting JP (2009) NLRP3 (NALP3, Cryopyrin) facilitates in vivo caspase-1 activation, necrosis, and HMGB1 release via

inflammasome-dependent and -independent pathways. J Immunol 183:2008–2015
10. Allen IC, Scull MA, Moore CB, Holl EK, McElvania-TeKippe E, Taxman DJ, Guthrie EH, Pickles RJ, Ting JP (2009) The NLRP3 inflammasome mediates in vivo innate immunity to influenza A virus through recognition of viral RNA. Immunity 30:556–565

Chapter 20

Intranasal Influenza Infection of Mice and Methods to Evaluate Progression and Outcome

Catherine J. Sanders, Brian Johnson, Charles W. Frevert, and Paul G. Thomas

Abstract

In vivo influenza infection models are critical for understanding viral dynamics and host responses during infection. Mouse models are extremely useful for infection studies requiring a high number of test animals. The vast array of gene knockout mice available is particularly helpful in investigating a particular gene's contributions to infection. Thus, more in vivo scientific experimentation of influenza has been done on mice than any other animal model. Here, we describe the technique of intranasal inoculation of mice and methods for assessing the severity of disease and humane endpoints, and discuss data acquired from infection of female C57BL/6J mice.

Key words Intranasal inoculation, influenza, 2,2,2-Tribromoethanol, Body weight loss, Animal euthanasia guidelines, Lung damage

1 Introduction

Influenza has dramatically impacted human populations. The 1918–1919 "Spanish" influenza epidemic resulted in roughly 50 million deaths worldwide [1, 2]. Subsequent pandemics in 1957 (H2N2 "Asian influenza") and 1968 (H3N2 "Hong Kong influenza") caused a reported 1.5–2 million and 1 million deaths, respectively [3–5]. The recent 2009 H1N1 pandemic, believed to cause relatively mild disease, has been found to have a global infection rate between 11 and 21 % and a case fatality rate of 0.03 % [6, 7]. Normal "seasonal" waves of influenza regularly result in over 30,000 deaths and 200,000 hospitalizations in the United States alone [8]. The continuing high number of severe cases demonstrates the need for further study on influenza pathogenesis. The host response to influenza, and the interplay of virus–host dynamics, is not particularly well understood and more work is needed.

Irving C. Allen (ed.), *Mouse Models of Innate Immunity: Methods and Protocols*, Methods in Molecular Biology, vol. 1031, DOI 10.1007/978-1-62703-481-4_20, © Springer Science+Business Media, LLC 2013

The advantages of using mice for in vivo studies are manifold. In comparison to other animal models used for influenza studies, breeding is quick and generally produces many offspring. As mice are an exceptionally well-studied species, their behavior in response to disease is well documented.

The genetic background of the host plays a critical role in the determination of susceptibility to a wide range of influenza isolates [9–11]. Mouse strains considered highly susceptible to influenza include A/J and DBA/2J [11, 12]. Strains considered moderately to minimally susceptible include Balb/C and C57BL/6J. Curiously, wild mice are resistant to some strains of influenza. This trait is attributed to the ability to synthesize Mx protein, an inducer of an antiviral state [13, 14]. Most inbred strains of mice have a functionally deleted Mx gene.

Influenza studies examining immunological memory responses frequently use a primary/secondary infection method, in which two different strains of virus are administered using the same or two different routes (for example, intranasally and intraperitoneally), separated by a specified period of time. Coinfection of influenza with bacteria or parasites generally follows a more complex administration protocol. Here, we describe a method for administration and evaluation of a primary influenza infection in C57BL/6 mice.

2 Materials

2.1 Infection

1. Virus diluted in 1× phosphate-buffered saline (PBS). Ensure that it is kept at 4 °C throughout preparation and administration. Select a virus concentration appropriate to the intention of the study (*see* **Note 1**).
2. 2,2,2-Tribromoethanol (Avertin) (*see* **Notes 2** and **3**).
3. Sterile 1 ml syringes and needles.
4. Positive displacement pipet.
5. Pistons.
6. Piston sheaths.

2.2 Noninvasive Evaluation: Weight Loss and Regain

1. Scale capable of weighing mice that range from 10 to 50 g.
2. Sided, flat-bottomed container that can fit on the weighing platform of the scale and can hold an active mouse without allowing for escape.

2.3 Invasive Evaluation: Plaque Assay on Madin–Darby Canine Kidney Cells

1. Confluent MDCK cells in 6-well plates (*see* **Note 4**) [15].
2. 37 °C incubator.
3. 37 °C water bath.
4. 65 °C water bath.

5. Vortex.
6. 6-Well plates.
7. Growth medium for MDCK cells (total volume 1 l): 100 ml of 10× MEM, 50 ml of fetal calf serum, 30 ml of 7.5 % sodium bicarbonate, 10 ml of penicillin/streptomycin (10,000 U/ml; 10,000 μg/ml), 10 ml of L-glutamine—200 mM (100×), 10 ml of MEM vitamin solution (100×), and 790 ml of ddH_2O.
8. Infection medium (total volume 1 l): 100 ml of 10× MEM, 40 ml of 7.5 % bovine serum albumin, 30 ml of 7.5 % sodium bicarbonate, 10 ml of penicillin/streptomycin (10,000 U/ml; 10,000 μg/ml), 10 ml of L-glutamine—200 mM (100×), 10 ml of MEM vitamin solution (100×), and 800 ml of ddH_2O.
9. 2× MEM medium (total 1 l): 200 ml of 10× MEM, 80 ml of 7.5 % bovine serum albumin, 60 ml of 7.5 % sodium bicarbonate, 20 ml of penicillin/streptomycin (10,000 U/ml; 10,000 μg/ml), 20 ml of L-glutamine—200 mM (100×), 20 ml of MEM vitamin solution (100×), and 600 ml of ddH_2O.
10. Tissue homogenizer.
11. Round-bottom polypropylene tubes able to hold minimum 2 ml volume (preferably 5 ml).
12. 1× PBS.
13. 200 μl and 1 ml pipettors.
14. TPCK trypsin (TPCK: L-(tosylamido-2-phenyl)ethyl chloromethyl ketone).
15. 1.8 % agar for overlay: 9 g Bacto-Agar, 500 ml sterile ddH_2O. Completely dissolve by heating, then autoclave.
16. Capped flask for mixing.
17. Tool, such as a spatula, for removing solidified agar overlay from 6-well plates.
18. Crystal violet staining reagent (1 l): 270 ml of 37 % formaldehyde solution, 730 ml of distilled H_2O, 1 g of crystal violet.

2.4 Invasive Evaluation: Lung Histology

1. Surgical tools (e.g., scissors, scalpel).
2. Syringe capable of holding 3 ml of fluid.
3. Thin catheter, able to fit in mouse trachea.
4. 10 % neutral buffered formalin solution.
5. Paraffin.
6. Device for sectioning tissues to 4 μm thickness.
7. Positively charged glass slides.
8. Hematoxylin and eosin stains.
9. Collagen stains Masson's Trichrome or Sirius Red, if desired.

3 Methods

3.1 Virus Dilution Method

1. Rapidly thaw aliquots of virus at 37 °C (*see* **Note 5**). Put the virus aliquots on ice immediately upon thawing.
2. Dilute the virus tenfold in ice-cold 1× PBS in polypropylene tubes and keep the virus on ice (*see* **Note 6**).
3. Keep the last dilution on ice throughout the duration of mouse infections.

3.2 Infection Method

1. Administer 2,2,2-tribromoethanol by intraperitoneal injection. Each animal should receive 250 mg/kg (*see* **Notes 7** and **8**).
2. Hold mice such that the head is tipped back and the nose is pointed upwards. Ensure that no pressure is exerted on the soft areas needed for nasal respiration (i.e., the nose and throat area) (Fig. 1).
3. Carefully expel virus through a positive displacement sheath/tip and droplets are put directly on the nostril openings. The mouse should inhale these droplets quickly. The speed of administration should match that of the mouse's inspiration of droplets.
4. Once the mouse has been inoculated, gently place the animal in an environment with mild heat and monitor until it regains consciousness (*see* **Note 9**).
5. If the experiment entails tracking the progress of infection of individual mice, then each mouse should be individually marked for identification (*see* **Note 10**).

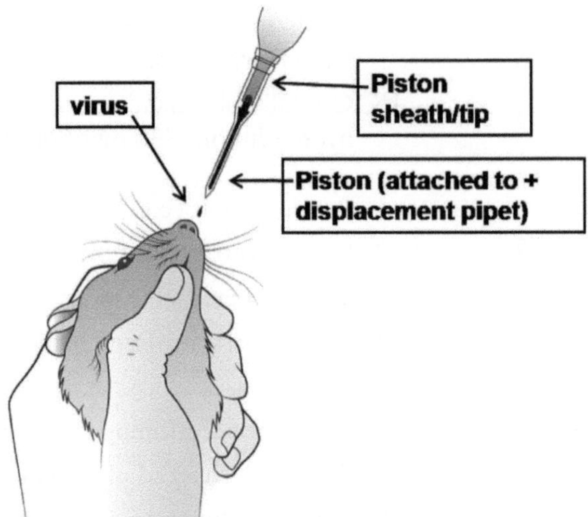

Fig. 1 Schematic illustrating the intranasal inoculation of virus to an anesthetized mouse

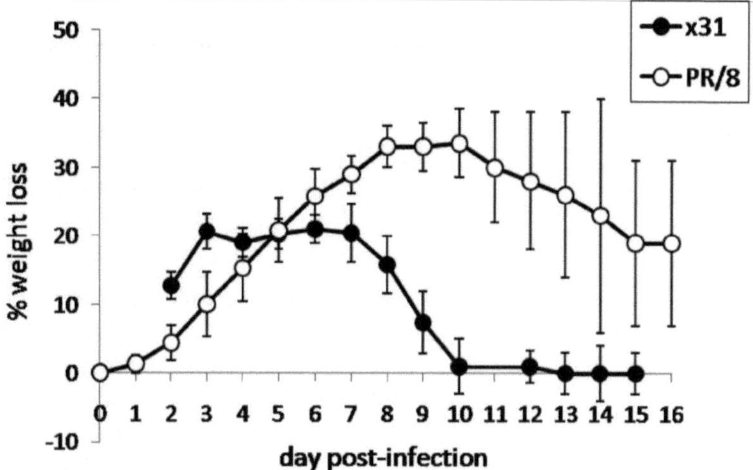

Fig. 2 Percent body weight loss kinetics of a nonlethal dose of ×31 (1×10^6 EID_{50}) to a dose of PR/8 that induces roughly half of C57BL/6 mice to meet our institutional guidelines for animal euthanasia (4×10^3 EID_{50}). ×31, $n = 20$ mice; PR/8, $n = 17$ mice. Eight days after infection, PR/8 infected mice are gradually euthanized. Standard deviation shown

3.3 Evaluation of Weight Loss and Regain

1. Monitor weight loss and recovery throughout the duration of the model (*see* **Note 11**). To evaluate weight, gently pick up the mouse by the base of the tail and transfer the animal to the container on the scale. Once a steady reading can be made, which is generally when the mouse has stopped moving around, record the weight. Ensure that a weight measurement has been taken for each mouse before the infection. This initial weight is necessary for the calculation of percent weight loss.
2. Calculate the percent weight change for each animal. Divide the difference of pre- versus postinfection weights and divide this difference by the pre-infection weight to obtain percent body weight change. Alternatively, divide postinfection body weight by baseline (pre-infection) body weight for each mouse to obtain the percent of original body weight. For example, weight loss curves over time of mice given a nonlethal dose of mouse-adapted influenza strain ×31 or a lethal dose of mouse-adapted strain PR/8 are shown in Fig. 2 (*see* **Notes 12–15**).

3.4 Viral Titer by Plaque Assay on MDCK Cells

1. One day before performing the plaque assay, seed an appropriate number of 6-well plates (one plate per six dilutions) with roughly 1.5×10^6 MDCK cells/well using 2 ml of infection medium/well. Keep overnight at 37 °C until use.
2. Homogenize each thawed lung in 2 ml of infection medium, and keep at 4 °C.
3. Prepare six tubes (select a size able to comfortably accommodate a 2 ml volume) for a tenfold serial dilution of each lung by adding 1.8 ml of infection medium/tube (*see* **Note 16**).

4. Set up the six tenfold dilutions of each virus. Briefly, add 200 μl of homogenized lung to the first tube and vortex. Continue this process for the remaining tubes.
5. Wash and prepare the MDCK-confluent plates. Briefly, aspirate the infection medium for each plate, and quickly replace with 3 ml of PBS. This is the first wash. Do three total washes per plate. Keep the cells on the last PBS wash until immediately before adding lung dilutions.
6. Add lung dilutions to the plates. Aspirate the last PBS wash, and then quickly add 1 ml of lung dilutions. Start by adding the lowest dilution to the last well of the 6-well plate, which allows for the addition of all dilutions without changing tips. Do not let the wells dry out.
7. Repeat this process for each plate.
8. Place the plates at 4 °C for 10 min.
9. Move the plates to 37 °C, and keep at this temperature for 50 additional minutes.
10. While the plates are incubating at 37 °C, prepare the agar overlay. Estimate 10 ml of 2× MEM per 6-well plate. Add enough 2× MEM for all plates to a capped flask and place in a 37 °C water bath. Next, add TPCK trypsin. You will need 20 μg per 10 ml of 2× MEM. The final step is to melt 1.8 % agar in a microwave. Once the agar is melted, place it in a 65 °C water bath to maintain its liquid state. You will need 10 ml of agar per 6-well plate.
11. After the plate incubation, remove 2× MEM and agar from the baths. Add TPCK trypsin to the 2× MEM then agar. For each 6-well plate, you will have 10 ml of 2× MEM, 10 μg of TPCK trypsin (1 μg/ml final concentration), and 10 ml of 1.8 % agar. Mix well without shaking.
12. Aspirate the liquid one plate at a time. Add 3 ml of 2× MEM/agar/TPCK trypsin mixture to each well, and repeat for each plate.
13. Allow the mixture to solidify on the plates for about 20 min.
14. Incubate at 37 °C for 72 h.
15. After incubation, carefully remove the solidified agar with a spatula. Do not scratch the bottom of the wells.
16. Add enough crystal violet to the wells to cover the bottom. Allow roughly 15 min for staining to occur.
17. Remove the crystal violet solution by a distilled water rinse.
18. Let the plates dry.
19. Count plaques and calculate the titer, keeping in mind the sequential tenfold dilutions of the lungs (*see* **Note 17**).

3.5 Lung Histology

1. Euthanize mouse on selected day after infection. Figures 5 and 6 show examples of lung histology on days 3 and 14 after infection, respectively (*see* **Notes 18** and **19**).
2. Gently inflate the lungs with 10 % neutral buffered formalin solution. This technique can be done via pushing the fluid through a syringe and an attached thin catheter inserted in a small hole in the trachea.
3. Surgically remove the whole lungs.
4. Immerse the infused tissue in the formalin for a minimum of 48 h.
5. Fix, paraffin embed, section (Figs. 5 and 6, tissues were sectioned at 4 μm), and mount the sections on positively charged glass slides.
6. Stain with hematoxylin and eosin (H&E). If visualization of collagen deposition is desired, stains such as Masson's Trichrome and Sirius Red allow for its detection. Figures 5 and 6 show examples of H&E and Sirius Red staining (*see* **Note 19**).
7. Evaluate lung histology.
8. Correlate the histologic evaluations with weight loss (*see* **Note 20**).

4 Notes

1. For infections to determine susceptibility, it is recommended to select a virus dose in the range of the LD_{50} of the particular virus stock. Figures 2, 3, and 4 show PR/8 doses ranging from 2×10^3 EID_{50} to 8×10^3 EID_{50} (50 % egg-infective dose).

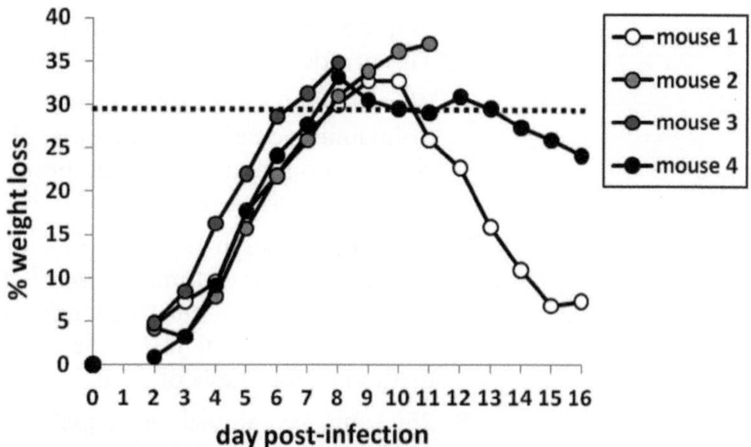

Fig. 3 Weight loss over time of individual C57BL/6 mice infected with 4×10^3 EID_{50} of mouse-adapted PR/8

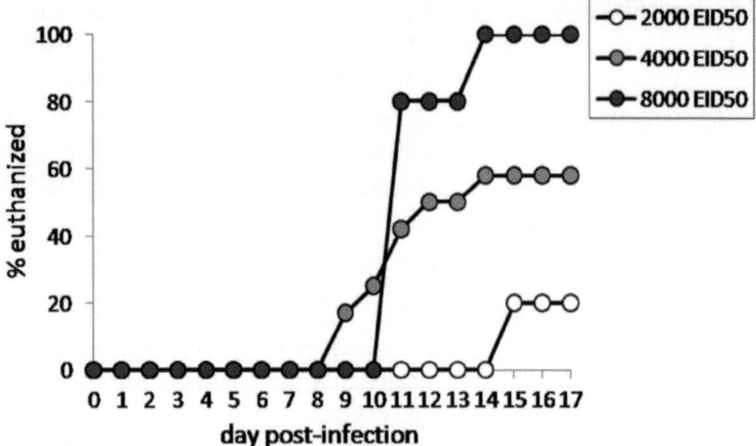

Fig. 4 Percentage of C57BL/6 mice meeting guidelines for euthanasia after PR/8 infection. 2×10^3 EID_{50}, $n = 5$ mice; 4×10^3 EID_{50}, $n = 12$ mice; 8×10^3 EID_{50}, $n = 5$ mice. All mice except one (in the 4×10^3 EID_{50} group) lost at least 30 % of their original body weight

2. Use of this anesthetic must be included on one's animal protocol, and must be approved by the institution's Institutional Animal Care and Use Committee (IACUC).
3. Protocols for the preparation of 2,2,2-tribromoethanol are widely available from numerous sources [16, 17]. Briefly, 0.5 g of 2,2,2-tribromoethanol is dissolved with heat and stirring per ml of 2-methyl-2-butanol. Distilled water is added to a final volume of 40 ml. This method results in a 12.5 mg/ml concentration. Sterile filter through a 0.2 μm filter. Protect from light and store at 4 °C.
4. The Madin–Darby canine kidney (MDCK) cell line is a highly utilized culture system for studying virus growth.
5. Aliquots of virus are generally kept at no more than 500 μl. This practice allows for rapid, thorough thawing.
6. We have found virus to be most stable at 4 °C. In our hands, maintaining consistent practices of keeping freshly thawed virus aliquots, and all virus dilutions, at ice-cold temperatures, gives reproducible in vivo (and in vitro) results.
7. 2,2,2-Tribromoethanol sedation will give approximately a 10-min window of time for inoculation. Isoflurane sedation, not described here but frequently used, provides about 10 s. A ketamine/xylazine injectable cocktail is another often used method of anesthesia of mice.
8. 250 mg/kg animal is equal to 0.4 ml of prepared 2,2,2-tribromoethanol solution per 20 g mouse.
9. Proper dosing with 2,2,2-tribromoethanol should lead to sedation within several minutes. The mouse should regain consciousness and the ability to right itself within 30–90 min.

10. Individual marking of mice may be done by a variety of methods, including but not restricted to metallic ear tag, ear notching, designated toe removal, tail marking, or tattooing. Most methods of uniquely identifying mice require proper animal protocol and IACUC approval.

11. The "gold standard" noninvasive method for evaluating morbidity in mice from influenza infection is the measurement of percentage weight loss. The technique is easily done as described in this protocol. Despite the widespread use of measuring mouse weight loss as a proxy for severity of infection, the method tells us little regarding physiological changes in the mouse. Body weight loss is in part a result of anorexia and lack of fluid intake, which presumably is a result of the mice feeling poor [18, 19].

12. Virus designations: PR/8: A/Puerto Rico/8/34 (PR8), H1N1. ×31: A/Aichi/02/68 (HA, NA)×A/Puerto Rico/8/34, H3N2.

13. Figure 2 demonstrates two clearly different weight loss curves as a result of infection with two different strains of influenza. Incidentally, the two strains of influenza only differ in their hemagglutinin (HA) and neuraminidase (NA). The nonlethal infection, ×31, induces a faster initial weight loss than the lethal PR/8 infection. Such patterns are presumably due to physiological responses to the higher viral load this group of mice received. However, weight loss of any individual mouse does not breech more than 25 % of the original weight. Mice infected with this dose of PR/8 exhibit a more gradual weight loss, yet ultimately reach, and in some cases surpass, 30 % loss of original body weight. Behaviors of mice at this point of infection, which we consider peak illness, include hunching, lack of grooming, and anorexia. Mice that become moribund as defined by our institutional protocols and body index scoring are euthanized. In this particular infection, about half of the mice reached this state. It is important to point out that about half the mice that reach the 30 % mark do not become moribund. In fact, they recover their body weights, demonstrating that body weight alone is a poor predictor of lethal outcome. The percent body weight loss of four example mice from the experiment shown in Fig. 2 are plotted individually in Fig. 3. Note the weight loss patterns of these four mice. Mouse 3 lost weight at an accelerated rate and became quickly moribund, while mice 1, 2, and 4 lost weight at comparable rates. However, only mouse 2 reached a state of illness requiring euthanasia. The other two recovered their body weights, albeit at different rates (Fig. 3).

14. The infectious dose generally dictates whether or not mice will reach a stage of illness requiring euthanasia. Comparison of percentage of mice meeting our institutional guidelines for

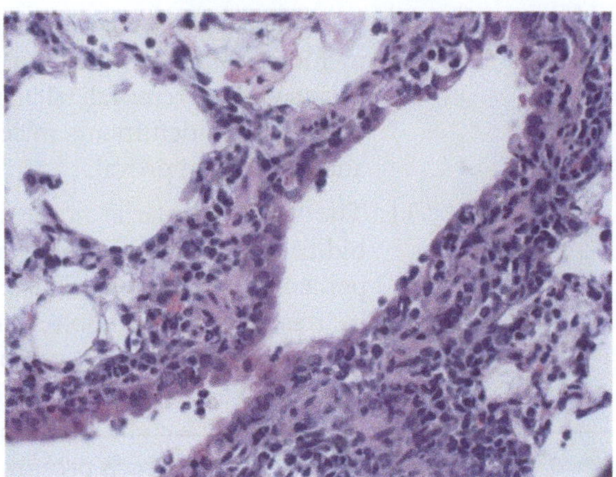

Fig. 5 C57BL/6 mouse lung histology 3 days after PR/8 infection. H&E stain shown at 400× magnification

sacrifice by PR/8 dose demonstrates this concept (Fig. 4). With the exception of one mouse that lost 27 %, all mice shown lost a minimum of 30 % of their original body weight. Here, 4/5 of mice receiving 2×10^3 EID_{50}, 5/12 mice in the 4×10^3 group, and 0/5 mice in the 8×10^3 EID_{50} group survived. Thus, care should be taken in infectious dose selection.

15. Tracking weight loss continues as a common measure of influenza progression. Guidelines for how much weight loss is considered acceptable (frequently including animal behavior) for continuing an in vivo animal infection experiment are often strictly set by an investigator's institution. It is becoming increasingly common to record humane endpoint euthanasia as "death by infection," but this should only be done if the humane endpoint serves as a relevant proxy for expected mortality. As shown, mice can lose at least 30 % of their original body weights and still recover, indicating that weight loss alone is not an appropriate proxy for death.
16. We have found 5 ml polypropylene tubes to work best for this purpose.
17. Infectious virus will form plaques, which when enumerated allows for the calculation of virus titer in the lungs. Units are recorded as plaque-forming units (PFU).
18. Extent and nature of cellular infiltration, tissue damage, and repair will vary by viral strain, initial viral load, and characteristics of the host animal.
19. Three days after the 4×10^3 EID_{50} PR/8 infection, the lungs exhibit focal necrosis of airway epithelium and a mild inflammatory response characterized by the presence of neutrophils, lymphocytes, and macrophages (Fig. 5). Figure 6 demonstrates

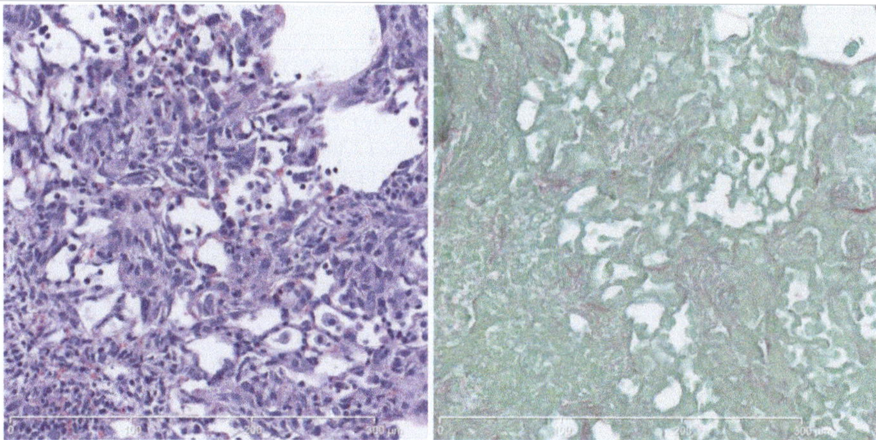

Fig. 6 C57BL/6 mouse lung histology 14 days after PR/8 infection. *Left*, H&E; *right*, Sirius Red

the type and degree of inflammation and damage seen in mouse lungs by day 14 after 4×10^3 EID_{50} PR/8 infection. At this later time, pneumonia was present in mice. Areas of active inflammation consisting of neutrophils, eosinophils, lymphocytes, and macrophages are present in the distal airways and the adjacent interstitium. Also in these locations, inflammation primarily composed of mononuclear cells is present. There is deposition of eosinophilic material here as well. Stains for collagen deposition, such as Masson's Trichrome and Sirius Red (Fig. 6, right), at this time point reveal a thin layer of collagen lining the alveolar spaces.

20. Though both weight loss and lung pathology are frequently used techniques for influenza disease evaluation, it is not well established how indicative the former is of the latter. Recently, a number of groups have published alternate methods for evaluation of the in vivo progress of influenza infection that correlate to lung pathology. These techniques, including pulse oximetry and plethysmography, appear promising in terms of prediction of susceptibility to infection [20, 21].

Acknowledgments

We would like to thank Betsy Williford and St. Jude Biomedical Communications for technical illustration, and Kelli Boyd and the St. Jude Veterinary Pathology core for histologic imaging and evaluation. This work was supported by NIAID contract number HHSN272200800058C.

References

1. Johnson NP, Mueller J (2002) Updating the accounts: global mortality of the 1918-1920 "Spanish" influenza pandemic. Bull Hist Med 76:105–115
2. Taubenberger JK, Morens DM (2006) 1918 Influenza: the mother of all pandemics. Emerg Infect Dis 12:15–22
3. Hilleman MR (2002) Realities and enigmas of human viral influenza: pathogenesis, epidemiology and control. Vaccine 20:3068–3087
4. Hsieh YC, Wu TZ, Liu DP, Shao PL, Chang LY, Lu CY, Lee CY, Huang FY, Huang LM (2006) Influenza pandemics: past, present and future. J Formos Med Assoc 105:1–6
5. Kilbourne ED (2006) Influenza pandemics of the 20th century. Emerg Infect Dis 12:9–14
6. Kelly H, Peck HA, Laurie KL, Wu P, Nishiura H, Cowling BJ (2011) The age-specific cumulative incidence of infection with pandemic influenza H1N1 2009 was similar in various countries prior to vaccination. PLoS One 6: e21828
7. LaRussa P (2011) Pandemic novel 2009 H1N1 influenza: what have we learned? Semin Respir Crit Care Med 32:393–399
8. Clark NM, Lynch JP III (2011) Influenza: epidemiology, clinical features, therapy, and prevention. Semin Respir Crit Care Med 32:373–392
9. Virelizier JL, Allison AC, Schild GC (1979) Immune responses to influenza virus in the mouse, and their role in control of the infection. Br Med Bull 35:65–68
10. Boon AC, Finkelstein D, Zheng M, Liao G, Allard J, Klumpp K, Webster R, Peltz G, Webby RJ (2011) H5N1 influenza virus pathogenesis in genetically diverse mice is mediated at the level of viral load. MBio 2:e00171–11
11. Srivastava B, Blazejewska P, Hessmann M, Bruder D, Geffers R, Mauel S, Gruber AD, Schughart K (2009) Host genetic background strongly influences the response to influenza a virus infections. PLoS One 4:e4857
12. Ding M, Lu L, Toth LA (2008) Gene expression in lung and basal forebrain during influenza infection in mice. Genes Brain Behav 7: 173–183
13. Haller O (1981) Inborn resistance of ice to orthomyxoviruses. Curr Top Microbiol Immunol 92:25–52
14. Haller O, Acklin M, Staeheli P (1987) Influenza virus resistance of wild mice: wild-type and mutant Mx alleles occur at comparable frequencies. J Interferon Res 7:647–656
15. Ho PP, Young AL, Truehaft M (1976) Plaque formation with influenza viruses in dog kidney cells. J Gen Virol 33:143–145
16. Cho YJ, Lee YA, Lee JW, Kim JI, Han JS (2011) Kinetics of proinflammatory cytokines after intraperitoneal injection of tribromoethanol and a tribromoethanol/xylazine combination in ICR mice. Lab Anim Res 27:197–203
17. Meyer RE, Fish RE (2005) A review of tribromoethanol anesthesia for production of genetically engineered mice and rats. Lab Anim (NY) 34:47–52
18. Swiergiel AH, Smagin GN, Dunn AJ (1997) Influenza virus infection of mice induces anorexia: comparison with endotoxin and interleukin-1 and the effects of indomethacin. Pharmacol Biochem Behav 57:389–396
19. Swiergiel AH, Smagin GN, Johnson LJ, Dunn AJ (1997) The role of cytokines in the behavioral responses to endotoxin and influenza virus infection in mice: effects of acute and chronic administration of the interleukin-1-receptor antagonist (IL-1ra). Brain Res 776:96–104
20. Julander JG, Hagloch J, Latimer S, Motter N, Dagley A, Barnard DL, Smee DF, Morrey JD (2011) Use of plethysmography in assessing the efficacy of antivirals in a mouse model of pandemic influenza A virus. Antiviral Res 92: 228–236
21. Verhoeven D, Teijaro JR, Farber DL (2009) Pulse-oximetry accurately predicts lung pathology and the immune response during influenza infection. Virology 390:151–156

Chapter 21

Dextran Sodium Sulfate-Induced Murine Inflammatory Colitis Model

Monika Schneider

Abstract

Colitis is a chronic inflammatory disease of the colon that is characterized by recurring, acute episodes. Mouse models of colitis allow for the study of multiple aspects of this disease, including the innate immune response, epithelial and intestinal cell response, and wound healing. The following protocols cover acute, chronic, and cancer-associated colitis models.

Key words IBD, Colon cancer, Inflammation-induced tumorigenesis, DSS, AOM, Azoxymethane

1 Introduction

Inflammatory bowel disease (IBD) is a chronic condition that requires a lifetime of care. Each year in the United States, $1.7 billion is spent on the treatment for this disease. Of the types of IBD, ulcerative colitis (UC) is one of the most prevalent. It is a chronic condition that affects up to 24 million people, including 1.4 million people in the United States [1]. Those individuals who have UC are more likely to go on to develop colorectal cancer, which is responsible for over 50,000 fatalities each year and is the fourth deadliest cancer in the United States [2]. Disease begins with an inflammatory insult, which damages the epithelial lining of the colon. This event leads to cellular infiltrate that is initially composed of macrophages and neutrophils, but can also include lymphocytes. These cells release cytokines and chemokines that attract additional leukocytes, increase vascular permeability, and lead to apoptosis of the local epithelial and crypt cells [3]. These cellular events can be manifested as loose and bloody stool. Inflammation causes thickening of the colon and inhibits uptake of nutrients and water. Repeated bouts of inflammation can lead to cellular dysplasia and hyperplasia, which eventually develop into tumors. This is especially true when the inflammation is coupled with genetic or environmental factors.

Irving C. Allen (ed.), *Mouse Models of Innate Immunity: Methods and Protocols*, Methods in Molecular Biology, vol. 1031, DOI 10.1007/978-1-62703-481-4_21, © Springer Science+Business Media, LLC 2013

Dextran sodium sulfate (DSS) is a detergent that becomes an irritant in the colon when ingested by mice. In this model of ulcerative colitis, DSS is included in the drinking water of mice and disease is driven by an innate immune response. The DSS will induce apoptosis of epithelial cells, which then leads to immune cell infiltration and exposes other cell types to the microbial flora. This inflammation is typically resolved 1–2 weeks after the DSS is removed from the drinking water. There are many parameters that can be measured in this model, including animal health via weight and clinical score, colon appearance and length, histological analysis of the colon, serum cytokines, proinflammatory cytokine expression, and inflammatory protein activation. The DSS model can be administered as an acute or a chronic model. It can also be used to induce inflammation that drives tumorigenesis in models of colitis-associated colon cancer (CAC).

2 Materials

1. Mice (male, strain C57Bl6, 7–10 weeks old) (*see* **Note 1**).
2. Dextran sodium sulfate (MP Pharmaceuticals; reagent grade, MW = 36,000–50,000) (*see* **Note 2**).
3. Scale for weighing mice.
4. Hemoccult fecal occult blood test.
5. 70 % ethanol.
6. Blunt-end scissors.
7. Curved forceps.
8. 26G Needles.
9. Tissue processing/histology cassettes (with slats for flow-through and resistant to chemicals).
10. 5 × 10 cm Whatman paper.
11. 10 % Formalin.
12. Liquid nitrogen.
13. 1 cm^3 syringes.
14. 5 cm^3 syringe.
15. PBS + 2× penicillin and streptomycin.
16. Optional: Azoxymethane (AOM) (Sigma).

3 Methods

3.1 Acute Colitis (See Note 3)

1. Separate mice into appropriate cages (*see* **Note 4**).
2. Make up the DSS solution by dissolving DSS in tap water (*see* **Note 5**).

3. On day 1, weigh the mice and replace drinking water with DSS water.
4. Weigh mice every day and note any change in fecal consistency, frequency, or rectal bleeding (*see* **Note 6**).
5. On day 5, remove the DSS water, rinse out the water bottle, and fill with tap water (*see* **Note 7**).
6. On day 8, assess a clinical score using the following parameters: stool consistency, blood in stool, and weight (*see* **Note 8**).
7. Harvest mice on day 14 (*see* **Note 9**).

3.2 Chronic Colitis

1. Separate mice into appropriate cages (*see* **Note 4**).
2. Make up the DSS solution by dissolving in tap water (*see* **Note 5**).
3. On day 1, weigh the mice and replace drinking water with 2–5 % DSS water.
4. Weigh mice every day and note any changes in fecal consistency, frequency, or rectal bleeding (*see* **Note 6**).
5. On day 5, remove the DSS water, rinse out the water bottle, and fill with tap water.
6. On day 8, assess a clinical score using the following parameters: stool consistency, blood in stool, and weight (*see* **Note 8**).
7. Weigh mice every other day.
8. Two weeks after replacing the DSS water with tap water, begin a second round of DSS treatment by replacing the tap water with DSS water, as described in Subheading 3.2, **steps 2** and **3** (*see* **Note 10**). Weigh mice every day for the next 5 days and note any diarrhea or rectal bleeding (*see* **Note 6**).
9. Five days after adding the DSS water, rinse out the water bottles and fill with tap water.
10. Two days after replacing the water, assess a clinical score (*see* **Note 8**).
11. Repeat Subheading 3.2, **steps 7–10**, for the third round of DSS.
12. Ten days after the removal of the DSS water, harvest the mice (*see* **Note 11**).

3.3 Colitis-Associated Colon Cancer

1. Prepare AOM at a 1:1,000 concentration (i.e., for 5 mL, add 5 μL of AOM).
2. Make up the DSS solution by dissolving in tap water (2–5 % depending on your experiment).
3. Separate mice into appropriate cages (*see* **Note 4**). For this model, the proper controls should include the following: mice that only drink tap water; mice that receive the AOM injection and only drink tap water; and mice that receive DSS treatments, but no AOM injection.

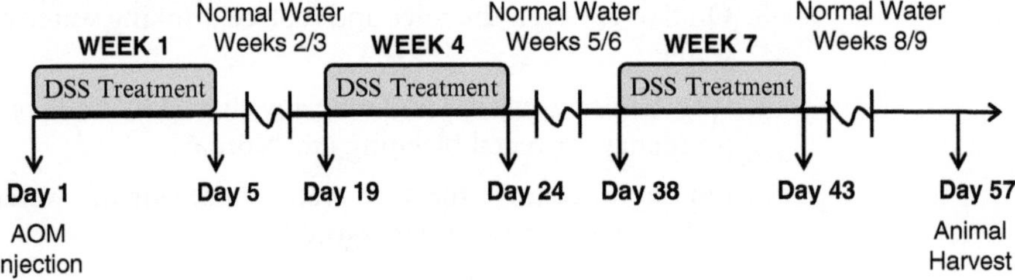

Fig. 1 Schematic for colitis-associated colon cancer model

4. Inject the appropriate control and experimental animals via intraperitoneal injection (i.p.) with 200 μL of AOM.
5. Follow **steps 3–12** outlined in Subheading 3.2 (Fig. 1).

3.4 Harvest

1. Euthanize mice using CO_2 asphyxiation.
2. Collect serum by cardiac puncture (*see* **Note 12**). After the serum has been collected from all of the mice, spin samples at maximum speed for 10 min. Remove the clear supernatant while avoiding red blood cell (RBC) aspiration and transfer to a new microcentrifuge tube. Discard the remaining RBCs and store serum samples at –80 °C.
3. Cut open the mouse from the rib cage to the base of the tail, being careful not to puncture the intestinal area. Remove the skin and pin to the sides of the animal.
4. Open the peritoneal cavity, being careful not to puncture the intestines.
5. If you are interested in assessing T or B cell function or numbers, or if you are interested in peripheral cytokine expression, remove the spleen and mesenteric lymph nodes. Take care to avoid damaging the intestines. For cell counts, cell culture, and flow cytometry, organs should be disrupted into a single-cell suspension. Cells and any lysates should be stored at –80 °C. For histology, organs should be placed into microcassettes and submerged in 10 % formalin solution.
6. Find the cecum. Remove the colon by cutting where it meets the cecum.
7. At the posterior of the mouse, remove the colon by cutting where it meets the rectum.
8. Gently remove the colon by pulling away connective tissue and lymph material.
9. Flush fecal matter from the colon (*see* **Note 13**).
10. Measure the length of the colon (*see* **Note 14**).
11. Lay the colon along Whatman paper. Moisten the area around the colon with PBS. Be careful to let the colon lay "naturally" on the filter paper and avoid stretching.

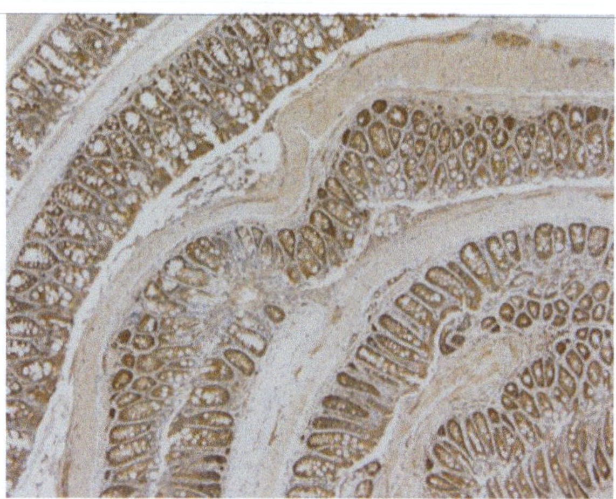

Fig. 2 H&E-stained histology image from a "Swiss roll" of the distal colon

12. Using blunt-end scissors and forceps, cut open the colon longitudinally.
13. If you are using the CAC model, identify, count, and measure macroscopic polyps (*see* **Note 15**).
14. If you are interested in gene expression or protein levels in the colon tissue, clip the most distal centimeter of colon, being careful to avoid any rectal tissue, and freeze in liquid nitrogen (*see* **Note 16**).
15. Roll the colon from the distal to the proximal end, forming a "Swiss roll" (Fig. 2).
16. Secure the Swiss roll by putting a needle through the center of the roll and transfer to a histology cassette. Place the cassette in 10 % formalin (*see* **Note 17**).

4 Notes

1. Severity of inflammation is dependent on the strain, age, and gender of the mouse. Typically, male mice are more susceptible than females. Mice under 6 weeks old will not have a fully developed immune system, and those that are older than 10 weeks will age out during the chronic model.
2. The proper molecular weight of DSS is necessary for development of disease.
3. Ensure that you have secured appropriate institutional approval before beginning animal experiments.
4. Because the DSS is in the drinking water, controls will need to be housed in separate cages. It is recommended that for each genotype tested, there is a group of each genotype that drinks

Table 1
Clinical score parameters

Weight loss (from baseline)	No weight loss or increase	0
	Weight loss of 1–5 %	1
	Weight loss of 6–10 %	2
	Weight loss of 11–20 %	3
	Weight loss of more than 20 %	4
Stool consistency	Well-formed pellets	0
	Semiformed stools (no anal adherence)	2
	Liquid stools (anal adherence)	4
Bleeding	No blood by hemoccult	0
	Positive hemoccult	2
	Gross bleeding	4

only water for the duration of the experiment. This setup will control for any baseline differences in weight.

5. Depending on the sensitivity of the genotype to DSS treatment, the percent of DSS can be adjusted. Typically 2–5 % DSS is used. For the acute model, a higher percentage of DSS is used (in our laboratory, we use 5 %). For chronic or CAC models, use a lower percentage of DSS (typically 2–3 %). The percent DSS is based on the total volume of the solution. For example, if one wanted 1 L of 3 % DSS, one would add 30 g of DSS to 1 L of tap water. The amount of water needed per cage of animals will vary with the number of animals in each cage and institutional regulations. In general, about 50 mL/cage/day is appropriate.
6. IACUC protocols dictate that animals that lose more than a stated percentage of body weight must be sacrificed. In our protocol, animals that maintain a 15–20 % weight loss over three measurements must be sacrificed.
7. Our experience suggests that tap water is necessary for the development of disease, and this step may be a source of variability.
8. Clinical score parameters are quantified using the scales described in Table 1.
9. Mice can be harvested at any point after day 12. The time between removal of DSS and harvest allows for colon repair, which decreases tearing of the colon during harvest.
10. If after 2 weeks the mice have not recovered from the first DSS treatment, then the recovery period should be extended by one additional week.
11. Mice can be harvested 7–14 days after the final round of DSS treatment.

12. We find this procedure to be most consistent when the mouse is pinned down on its back, with each foot pulled away from the body. The needle should be inserted 5 mm to the right and 5 mm up from the base of the sternum.

13. To flush the colon, we recommend using 1× PBS with 2× penicillin and streptomycin added. Wrap a thin strip of parafilm around the nozzle of a 10 cm^3 syringe. Fill the syringe with PBS/antibiotics. Place an unfiltered 200 μL tip on the end of the syringe. Wrap the base of the tip with parafilm to create an airtight seal. The tip can then be placed in the proximal end of the colon, and colon and tip held with forceps, to flush fecal matter.

14. Colon length is used as a surrogate assessment for inflammation. If the colon is inflamed, it will shorten in length and become thicker.

15. Phenotypic differences in the CAC model are partially determined by differences in the number and size of polyps. Location (distal vs. proximal) of the polyps may also provide clues to the mechanism of disease.

16. This piece of tissue can be homogenized in the appropriate buffer to extract protein or RNA for analysis.

17. The roll can be sliced to maximize surface area, showing a cross section of the entire colon, at a thickness of 5 μm. Damage to the colon can be identified using H&E staining.

References

1. Lakatos P-L (2006) Recent trends in the epidemiology of inflammatory bowel diseases: up or down? World J Gastroenterol 12(38): 6102–6108
2. 1999–2007 Cancer Incidence and Mortality Data. Center for Disease Control and Prevention. http://apps.nccd.cdc.gov/uscs/. Downloaded 12/14/2012
3. Terzić J, Grivennikov S, Karin E, Karin M (2010) Inflammation and colon cancer. Gastroenterology 138(6):2101.e5–2114.e5

Chapter 22

Bacterial Mediated Gastrointestinal Inflammation

Joshua Uronis and Xiaolun Sun

Abstract

Mouse models have proven to be a key approach in our understanding of the etiology and physiology underlying bacterial mediated gastrointestinal inflammation. Generally, these models are based on the inoculation of genetically susceptible mice with either commensal or pathogenic bacteria to elicit an inflammatory response. Here, we describe models of acute and chronic gastrointestinal inflammation using interleukin 10-deficient (*Il10*$^{-/-}$) mice colonized with the pathogenic *Campylobacter jejuni* strain 81-176 or the commensal *Escherichia coli* strain NC 101.

Key words Gastrointestinal inflammation, *Il10*$^{-/-}$ mouse, *Campylobacter jejuni*, *Escherichia coli*

1 Introduction

The human colon serves as a host for tens of thousands of bacterial species. It is estimated that these bacteria number into the hundreds of trillions [1, 2]. These diverse bacterial communities benefit by occupying their host who provides a source of nutrients. The host in turn derives physiological benefits provided by the bacteria [2]. Commensal bacteria have been found to play a direct role in biological processes including development of the mucosal immune system and nutrient metabolism [3]. Although we derive significant benefit from the presence of the gut microbiota, under certain circumstances the relationship between bacteria and human can go awry [4]. It is now well established that the gut microbiota plays a role in the etiology of chronic inflammatory bowel diseases, such as Crohn's disease and ulcerative colitis [5], although the mechanisms underlying these processes remain to be elucidated.

In addition to understanding the role of commensal bacteria in physiology and chronic diseases of the gut, of significant importance is the investigation of mechanisms underlying acute gastrointestinal infection by pathogenic bacteria. Gastrointestinal enteritis induced by pathogenic bacteria is a major threat worldwide. Annually, millions of people are infected every year with food- and

Irving C. Allen (ed.), *Mouse Models of Innate Immunity: Methods and Protocols*, Methods in Molecular Biology, vol. 1031, DOI 10.1007/978-1-62703-481-4_22, © Springer Science+Business Media, LLC 2013

waterborne bacterial pathogens, including *Campylobacter jejuni*, *Salmonella Typhimurium*, and certain strains of *Escherichia coli* [6, 7]. Billions of dollars are spent annually on efforts aimed at the prevention and treatment of these diseases. Despite the prevalence of pathogenic gastroenteritis worldwide, we still have a limited view as to the mechanisms underlying bacterial pathogenesis. This limited view is partly due to a lack of appropriate models with which to study these processes.

As part of ongoing research to identify mechanisms by which bacteria promote gastrointestinal disease, mouse models of bacterial induced colitis have been established [8, 9]. The development of technologies including germfree/gnotobiotic and gene knockout mice has been integral to this process [8]. The combination of these technologies has allowed us to model the behavior of the gut under conditions that closely recapitulate those found in patients with inflammatory bowel diseases, as well as acute conditions such as pathogen-induced gastroenteritis [9–11].

A predominant model used in the investigation of bacterial mediated gut inflammation is established by inoculating a genetically compromised host, commonly the germfree *Il10*$^{-/-}$ mouse, with either pathogenic or commensal (nonpathogenic) bacteria [12].

2 Materials

2.1 Animals

1. *Il10*$^{-/-}$ 129/SvJ mice under germfree (GF) or specific pathogen-free (SPF) housing between 8 and 12 weeks of age (*see* **Note 1**).
2. Provide mice a standard chow diet and water *ad libitum*.

2.2 Bacteria

1. *C. jejuni*: strain 81-176.
2. *E. coli*: strain NC 101.

2.3 Culture Materials

1. *C. jejuni*: Mueller Hinton agar, *Campylobacter* selective blood plates (Remel), Columbia broth.
2. *E. coli*: Lysogeny Broth (LB) agar and LB liquid broth.
3. GasPak Jar (GasPak EZ Campy container system).
4. Petri dishes.
5. L-shape cell spreaders.
6. Inoculation loops.
7. Cell scrapers.

2.4 Antibiotics

1. Streptomycin.
2. Gentamicin.
3. Bacteriocin.
4. Ciprofloxacin.

2.5 Gavage Instruments

1. PS20 gavage needles.
2. 1 ml syringes.

2.6 Other Materials

1. Spectrophotometer.
2. Cuvettes.
3. Pipettes: 20; 200; and 1,000 μl.
4. Pipette tips: 20; 200; and 1,000 μl.

3 Methods

3.1 Antibiotic Treatment for SPF Mice (Not Required for GF Mice)

1. Prepare the following antibiotic cocktail: Streptomycin 2 g/L, bacteriocin 1 g/L, gentamicin. 0.5 g/L, and ciprofloxacin 0.125 g/L in distilled water.
2. Stir the solution at room temperature until all antibiotics dissolve.
3. Provide mice with antibiotic cocktail in place of their drinking water.
4. Replace the cocktail every 2 days with a freshly made stock.
5. After 7 days of antibiotic treatment, transfer the mice to clean cages.

3.2 C. jejuni Infection

1. Two days before *C. jejuni* infection, pipette 70 μl of *C. jejuni* stock on *C. jejuni*-selective blood plates and spread the bacteria using an L-shape cell spreader.
2. Place the plates into a GasPak EZ Campy container system at 37–42 °C for 2 days with 1 gas-generating sachet. *C. jejuni* grows optimally under microaerobic conditions, specifically 85 % N_2, 10 % CO_2, and 5 % O_2.
3. Collect the top layer of *C. jejuni* from the plates and transfer into Columbia broth using a cell scraper.
4. Measure the optical density (OD_{600}) of the *C. jejuni* in Columbia broth to generate an estimate of colony-forming units (CFU).
5. Hold mice firmly and orally gavage 200 μl of Columbia broth containing ~5×10^9 CFU/ml of *C. jejuni* (10^9 CFU) per mouse.

3.3 E. coli Infection

1. Streak *E. coli* NC 101 on an LB plate.
2. Place the plate at 37 °C in an aerobic incubator overnight.
3. After colonies have formed, pick one colony into LB broth and incubate at 37 °C with shaking overnight at 250–300 rpm.
4. After overnight incubation, spin down the culture at $200 \times g$ and resuspend the pellet in fresh LB broth.

Table 1
Score system for evaluating colonic inflammation using H&E tissue slides

Inflammation score	Histopathological features
0	No immune cell infiltration No epithelial hyperplasia Presence of goblet cells
1	Infiltrating small number of immune cells into focal or partial lamina propria Minimal epithelial hyperplasia Presence of goblet cells
2	Infiltrating extensive immune cells into partial lamina propria Obvious epithelial hyperplasia Mild loss of goblet cells
3	Infiltrating profound immune cells into entire lamina propria Marked epithelial hyperplasia Moderate to marked loss of goblet cells Crypt architecture distortion
4	Crypt abscesses Crypt ulcerations Transmural inflammation Absence of crypts

5. Measure the OD_{600} of the *E. coli* culture to estimate CFU (*see* **Note 2**).
6. Hold mice firmly and gavage 200 μl of 5×10^8 CFU/ml *E. coli* (1×10^8) per mouse.

3.4 Evaluating Intestinal Inflammation

1. *C. jejuni*-induced intestinal inflammation may be assessed 2 weeks post infection in germfree *Il10*$^{-/-}$ mice and in 2–4 weeks in antibiotic-treated SPF mice.
2. *E. coli*-induced intestinal inflammation may be evaluated 4 weeks post infection in germfree *Il10*$^{-/-}$ mice.
3. At the end of the experiment, euthanize mice using CO_2 asphyxiation (*see* **Note 3**).
4. Swiss roll preparation: Remove the colon, flush out the stool with PBS, and splay the colon longitudinally on a piece of Whatman filter paper. Roll the colon beginning from the distal to the proximal end so that it resembles a Swiss roll. Secure the roll with a 27–30 gauge needle to keep it from unraveling.
5. Fix the colon in 10 % buffered formalin overnight at 4 °C and process for H&E histological evaluation.
6. If desired, collect colon, mesenteric lymph node, and spleen tissues for further processing for RNA, protein, or bacterial culture.

7. If desired, process blank tissue slides to visualize bacterial invasion into the colon by fluorescence in situ hybridization.
8. Intestinal inflammation is assessed in H&E histology slides based on the degree of lamina propria immune cell infiltration, goblet cell depletion, architectural distortion, crypt hyperplasia, ulceration, and abscesses using a standard score from 0 to 4 (Table 1).

4 Notes

1. This model has been tested with C57BL/6 and 129/SvJ mice. C57BL/6 mice are more resistant to bacterial induced colitis using this model under most housing conditions; therefore, it is suggested that 129/SvJ mice be used in this model.
2. Generally, an OD_{600} reading of 1 equals $2–8 \times 10^8$ CFU/ml *E. coli.*
3. It is necessary to seek permission from all relevant animal regulatory bodies (i.e., IACUC) prior to beginning experiments. Note that methods of euthanasia vary between institutions. Be sure to use the methods authorized by your institution.

Acknowledgments

We would like to acknowledge Ryan Balfour Sartor M.D. and Dr. Christian Jobin Ph.D. in the Center for Gastrointestinal Biology and Disease at the University of North Carolina at Chapel Hill for establishing these protocols through their research efforts in the investigation of bacterial induced intestinal epithelial inflammation.

References

1. Frank DN, St Amand AL, Feldman RA, Boedeker EC, Harpaz N, Pace NR (2007) Molecular-phylogenetic characterization of microbial community imbalances in human inflammatory bowel diseases. Proc Natl Acad Sci U S A 104(34):13780–13785
2. Neish AS (2009) Microbes in gastrointestinal health and disease. Gastroenterology 136(1):65–80
3. Turnbaugh PJ, Ley RE, Hamady M, Fraser-Liggett CM, Knight R, Gordon JI (2007) The human microbiome project. Nature 449(7164):804–810
4. Haller D, Jobin C (2004) Interaction between resident luminal bacteria and the host: can a healthy relationship turn sour? J Pediatr Gastroenterol Nutr 38(2):123–136
5. Mantovani A (2005) Cancer: inflammation by remote control. Nature 435(7043):752–753
6. Scallan E, Hoekstra RM, Angulo FJ, Tauxe RV, Widdowson MA, Roy SL, Jones JL, Griffin PM (2011) Foodborne illness acquired in the United States–major pathogens. Emerg Infect Dis 17(1):7–15
7. Blaser MJ (1997) Epidemiologic and clinical features of Campylobacter jejuni infections. J Infect Dis 176(Suppl 2):S103–S105
8. Sellon RK, Tonkonogy S, Schultz M, Dieleman LA, Grenther W, Balish E, Rennick DM, Sartor RB (1998) Resident enteric bacteria are

necessary for development of spontaneous colitis and immune system activation in interleukin-10-deficient mice. Infect Immun 66(11):5224–5231

9. Lippert E, Karrasch T, Sun X, Allard B, Herfarth HH, Threadgill D, Jobin C (2009) Gnotobiotic IL-10; NF-kappaB mice develop rapid and severe colitis following Campylobacter jejuni infection. PLoS One 4(10):e7413

10. Sun X, Threadgill D, Jobin C (2012) Campylobacter jejuni induces colitis through activation of mammalian target of rapamycin signaling. Gastroenterology 142(1):86–95.e85

11. Patwa LG, Fan TJ, Tchaptchet S, Liu Y, Lussier YA, Sartor RB, Hansen JJ (2011) Chronic intestinal inflammation induces stress-response genes in commensal Escherichia coli. Gastroenterology 141(5):1842–1851, e1841–1810

12. Kim SC, Tonkonogy SL, Karrasch T, Jobin C, Sartor RB (2007) Dual-association of gnotobiotic IL-10$^{-/-}$ mice with 2 nonpathogenic commensal bacteria induces aggressive pancolitis. Inflamm Bowel Dis 13(12):1457–1466

Chapter 23

Plasmodium berghei ANKA (PbA) Infection of C57BL/6J Mice: A Model of Severe Malaria

Marcela Montes de Oca, Christian Engwerda, and Ashraful Haque

Abstract

The term "severe malaria" refers to a wide spectrum of syndromes in *Plasmodium*-infected humans including cerebral malaria (CM), respiratory distress, severe anemia, liver dysfunction, and hypoglycemia. Mouse models have been employed to further our understanding of the pathology and immune responses that occur during *Plasmodium* infection. Evidence of brain, liver, lung, and spleen pathology, as well as anemia and tissue-sequestration of parasites, has been reported in various strains of inbred mice. While no single mouse model mimics all the various clinical manifestations of severe malaria in humans, here we describe a detailed protocol for *Plasmodium berghei* ANKA infection of C57BL/6J mice. For many years, this model has been referred to as "experimental cerebral malaria," but in fact recapitulates many of the symptoms and pathologies observed in most severe malaria syndromes.

Key words Mouse models, Malaria, *Plasmodium*, Blood-stage, Disease, Experimental cerebral malaria, Pathology

1 Introduction

Mouse models of malaria have been employed for many years to establish how *Plasmodium*/host molecular interactions result in disease, and to define possible mechanisms for, and obstacles against, the generation of anti-*Plasmodium* immunity in humans. It is argued here that such methods in mice complement clinical, epidemiological, and genetic approaches undertaken in humans.

Various mouse models have been used to model lethal and nonlethal malaria, usually involving infection of inbred mouse strains with rodent-infective *Plasmodium* species such as *P. chabaudi*, *P. yoelii*, *P. vinckei*, and *P. berghei* [1–5]. Within the *P. berghei* species there are various strains that have been used experimentally, including *P. berghei* ANKA (PbA). The PbA genome was sequenced in 2005 [6], and given that transfection methods have also been developed for this strain [7, 8], it has become an attractive choice for malaria parasite biologists.

Irving C. Allen (ed.), *Mouse Models of Innate Immunity: Methods and Protocols*, Methods in Molecular Biology, vol. 1031, DOI 10.1007/978-1-62703-481-4_23,

For example, a recently launched open resource, called PlasmoGem, hosted by the Wellcome Trust Sanger Institute, Hinxton, Cambridge, UK (http://www.sanger.ac.uk), will be a vector resource for the generation of gene-specific knockout PbA parasites.

It has been established now for more than 20 years in various laboratories worldwide that a severe, ultimately fatal disease is induced in PbA-infected C57BL/6J mice [9–11]. The most severe symptoms of this disease in mice appear to be neurologically related, with evidence of motor dysfunction, fitting, and/or coma [1, 12]. It is when neurological symptoms are observed in these mice that local ethics committees require them to be humanely euthanized. It is interesting to note that even if mice can be cured of their neurological symptoms, long-term cognitive impairment has been reported [13, 14].

Given that neurological symptoms appear to be fatal in PbA-infected C57BL/6J mice, research has focused on the study of brain pathology. Numerous studies have demonstrated inflammation within the brain, including breakdown of the blood–brain barrier (BBB) [15], and upregulation of inflammatory markers such as ICAM-1 and VCAM-1 on brain endothelial cells [16]. An important role for immune-pathology has been elucidated in the brain, with hundreds of thousands of parasite-specific $CD8^+$ cytotoxic T cells migrating to the brain, and causing death via perforin/granzyme B-dependent mechanisms [17–19]. The exact target of these $CD8^+$ T cells remains unclear, although brain endothelial cells are possible candidates. It is interesting to note that visualizing these cells by microscopic analysis of murine brain tissue sections is notoriously difficult due to their low frequency [20]. It has been through the use of cell isolation techniques and flow cytometric analyses that a role for T cell immune pathology was elucidated in mice.

In addition to brain pathology, it has become increasingly clear in recent years that PbA infection causes widespread pathology in other organs. Various reports provide convincing evidence of acute lung pathology and associated respiratory distress in PbA infection in various inbred mouse strains [21–23]. Metabolic acidosis is a major feature of severe malaria in humans, and this too is observed in PbA-infected mice [24]. Liver damage is also a feature of severe malaria in humans, which can be reversed by clearance of the parasite [25]. This observation has been mirrored in PbA infection of C57BL/6J mice [26].

The pathogenesis of severe malaria syndromes in humans remains unclear, but is thought to rely on the adherence of parasitized red blood cells (pRBCs) in the microvasculature of various tissues, a process known as "sequestration" [27, 28]. In humans, malaria disease severity correlates strongly with the total number of parasites within the body, i.e., the sum of those circulating freely in the bloodstream and those sequestered in tissues [29]. Recently, PbA-infected C57BL/6J mice have been studied in this context. Using transgenic, biomarker-expressing parasites, it appears that pRBCs accumulate in many different tissues in PbA-infected C57BL/6J mice, including the lung, liver, spleen, and brain, and that the total number of parasites in the body accurately predicts disease severity [10, 11, 17, 30].

Given all the evidence above, we argue here that PbA infection of C57BL/6J mice provides an excellent model to study numerous aspects of severe malaria in humans. Thus, we describe a detailed protocol for PbA infection of C57BL/6J mice. We use a dose of 10^5 pRBC injected intravenously (i.v.) via a lateral tail vein. Various other infection regimens are common in the scientific literature, including dosing with 10^6 pRBC intraperitoneally, or 10^4 pRBC i.v. [31, 32]. The choice of which regimen to use is perhaps a relatively minor consideration since all of these trigger severe and fatal symptoms in C57BL/6J mice. Nevertheless, we acknowledge that larger inoculum sizes may trigger quantitatively and qualitatively different host responses in comparison to much smaller inocula.

Using a 10^5 pRBC dose i.v., at approximately 5 days post infection (p.i.) mice exhibit mild symptoms such as ruffled fur, lethargy, and hunching. However, within a further 24–48 h more severe neurological symptoms such as convulsions, limb paralysis, and coma are observed [1]. Approximately 90–95 % of mice are euthanized due to neurological symptoms between 6 and 10 days p.i., with a small minority of mice surviving [1]. It is important to note that mice which have survived the window of severe neurological symptoms between days 6 and 10 p.i. will still become moribund around 20 days p.i, when they display evidence of anemia and hyperparasitemia [1]. These mice must also be euthanized according to guidelines from a local ethics committee.

Ethics approval must be obtained from a local institutional ethics committee prior to the commencement of any experiments with this model. PbA is a rodent-specific *Plasmodium* species and is therefore not infectious towards humans. However, all necessary precautions and risk assessment procedures must be strictly adhered to. The major procedures involved in this protocol include aseptic techniques, intravenous and intraperitoneal (i.p.) injections, and standard light microscopy.

2 Materials

2.1 Equipment

1. Sterilized carbon steel surgical blades.
2. Microscope slides.
3. 1 mL Insulin syringes with 27″ needle.
4. 1 mL Injection syringes with 26″ needles.

5. 10 mL polypropylene conical tubes.
6. 50 mL polypropylene conical tubes.
7. Pasteur pipettes.
8. Hemocytometer (0.0025 mm^2).
9. Light microscope (e.g., Olympus CXC31—use ×100 oil objective).
10. Inverted light microscope (e.g., Olympus CKX41—10× objective required).
11. Giemsa-based stains.
12. 3× vertical staining jars (58 mm × 53.5 mm × 86 mm).
13. Pipettes: P1000; P200; P20; P10; and tips.
14. 96 U-well bottom plate.
15. Freezing container (−1°/min).
16. Isopropanol.
17. 1 mL Cryo NUNC vials.
18. C57BL/6J mice, female, aged 6–8 weeks.

2.2 Preparation of Media and Reagents

1. Roswell Park Memorial Institute (RPMI) media.
2. 10× Penicillin and streptomycin (PenStrep): 10,000 U/mL Penicillin and 10,000 μg/mL streptomycin. PenStrep are antibiotics used to prevent bacterial contamination of cell cultures due to their effective action against gram-positive and gram-negative bacteria, respectively. Aliquot 10 mL of 10× PenStrep into 10 mL polypropylene conical tubes. There should be enough for ten tubes. Use one tube for the current experiments and store the remaining tubes at −20 °C.
3. Heparin (5,000 IU/mL).
4. 1 % Biodyne diluted in water (for waste disposal).
5. Glycerol.
6. Fetal calf serum.
7. Trypan blue stock solution: 0.4 % solution in 1× PBS.
8. 0.1 % Trypan blue working solution: Dilute the 0.4 % Trypan blue stock solution 1:4 in 1× PBS.
9. RPMI/PS media: Add 5 mL of PenStrep to 495 mL of fresh RPMI media.
10. 6. pRBC freezing medium: 15 % glycerol, 5 % FCS, RPMI.

For example: For a packed cell volume (PCV) of 2 mL, the amount of freezing medium needed will be two times the PCV (2× PCV = 4 mL). Therefore the freezing medium will contain 15 % glycerol (4,000 μl × 0.15 = 600 μL of glycerol), 5 % FCS (4,000 μl × 0.05 = 200 μL of FCS), and RPMI (4,000 μL (total volume) − 800 μL (volume already added) = 3.2 mL of RPMI).

3 Methods

3.1 In Vivo Passage of Parasites

1. Obtain a PbA stabilate from a collaborating laboratory (approximately 0.2–0.5 mL with 1–5 % parasitemia, when frozen down) and keep in liquid nitrogen until required. This preparation contains pRBC in a glycerol-rich (15 % v/v) medium to minimize cell-lysis. Of the various *Plasmodium* life-cycle stages in the blood, it is only the more robust "ring" stages that survive this freeze–thaw process. Thus, preparations containing mostly late-stage schizonts, for example, will not survive well in stabilates.
2. When required, defrost the vial of PbA stabilate (using the heat of your gloved hand is sufficient).
3. Take up the stabilate into a 1 mL syringe loaded with a 26 or a 27G needle (which should have minimum "dead volume"). We suggest using a "27G Terumo insulin syringe" where the needle and syringe body are fixed together, and the dead volume is small. Inject the stabilite into a C57BL/6J mouse intraperitoneally.
4. pRBC should be detectable by blood smear from day 3 or 4 post inoculation onwards. We suggest checking parasitemia from day 3 onwards, and to harvest blood for setting up infection when parasitemia is between 1 and 4 %. The protocol for performing blood smears is below.

3.2 Determination of Peripheral Blood Parasitemia

1. Using a sterile scalpel, cut <1 mm from the tip of tail of the mouse.
2. Run thumb and index fingers along the left and right lateral veins of the tail to milk a small drop of blood and collect onto a labeled glass slide, approximately 1/3 the distance of the glass surface away from the labeled area.
3. Working quickly to avoid the blood drying out, place the slide with the drop of blood onto a flat surface and use an additional clean slide (the "smearing" slide) to spread the blood drop evenly across the slide surface to create a thin layer of blood. This is done by holding the smearing slide at an acute angle relative to the flat slide, and dragging it back until the drop of blood forms a red line against the interface between the two slides. When this has occurred, push the smearing slide smoothly along the flat slide, ensuring that firm contact between the two slides is maintained (Fig. 1).
4. Allow the slide to fully dry before soaking the slide in fixative solution for 2 min (*see* **Note 1**).
5. Blot the edge of the slide (leaving the smear untouched) on an absorbent tissue before soaking in counterstain #1 for 1 min.

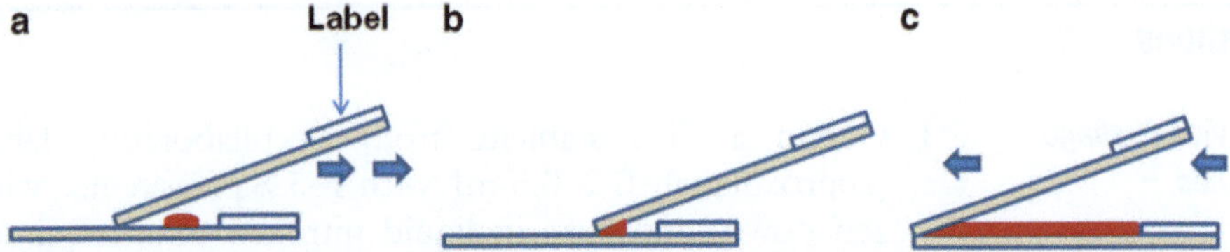

Fig. 1 Preparation of blood smears. (**a**) Milk a drop of blood and collect onto a labeled glass slide. (**b**) Use an additional slide angled at 45° to draw the slide back up to the drop of blood, forming a line of blood across the slide surface. (**c**) Gently push the slide forward so that a thin layer of blood is visible across the slide surface. Images courtesy of Shannon Best

6. Finally, after blotting the side of the slide on the tissue, soak the slide in counterstain #2 for 2 min. Run tap water over the slide for 10–15 s to wash.
7. Once the slide is completely dry, examine under a standard light microscope using a 100× oil immersion objective. A drop of oil can be placed directly onto the smear without the need of a coverslip. This will not damage the smear. The oil can be dabbed off at anytime using Kim wipes, and the slide stored at room temperature indefinitely.
8. Scan through the slide and select an area where RBCs are visible as a monolayer (ensure that there is no or minimal overlapping of RBC).
9. Count a minimum of 1,000 RBCs and determine the percentage of cells that are pRBC positive. We suggest spreading this count over multiple, well-separated fields of view to normalize for local variations in parasitization that occur in the smear.

3.3 Preparation of pRBCs for Infection

1. Perform all of the following steps in a class II biosafety hood.
2. Aliquot 5 mL of RPMI/PS and 5 μL of heparin into a 10 mL polypropylene conical tube.
3. Euthanize the passage mouse in accordance with local ethics committee guidelines, for example, via CO_2 asphyxiation, cervical dislocation, or other methods.
4. Perform a cardiac bleed, to obtain as much blood as possible (500–800 μL optimal) using an insulin syringe. Transfer to the 5 mL of RPMI/PS + heparin-containing media and gently mix well by inverting the tube up and down five times (*see* **Note 2**).
5. Bring the volume up to 10 mL, by adding approximately 5 mL of RPMI/PS.
6. Centrifuge cells at 1,127 ×*g* for 7 min at room temperature.
7. Carefully (because the red blood cell pellet is loose) aspirate the supernatant using a Pasteur pipette and resuspend the pellet in 1 mL of RPMI/PS (*see* **Note 3**).
8. Perform an accurate count of the concentration of red blood cells in the preparation. Since it is a concentrated preparation,

with approximately one billion red blood cells per mL, it is necessary to dilute the blood for counting, as detailed below.

9. From the concentrated blood preparation make a 1:1,000 dilution (e.g., add 10 μL of concentrated preparation to 10 mL of RPMI/PS, and mix well by repeated tube inversion).
10. From the 1,000-fold diluted sample, perform a 1:2 dilution into 0.1 % Trypan blue (e.g., add 50 μL of 1:1,000 dilution mixture to 50 μL of 0.1 % Trypan blue in a single well of a 96-well, round-bottomed plate).
11. Load 10 μL of the 1:2 dilution mixture into the chamber of a hemocytometer. Since such a small volume is being loaded onto the hemocytometer, ensure that each sample is well mixed by pipetting, prior to loading.
12. Using the 10× objective on an inverted light microscope, count total red blood cells.
13. The dose used in this protocol is 10^5 pRBC injected i.v. However, please note that others have used inoculum ranging from 10^4 to 10^6 pRBC, although the route of administration may vary in other reports.
14. Once the inoculum has been prepared, inject 200 μL i.v. into mice within 2 h.

3.4 Making PbA Stabilate Stocks

1. Perform all of the following steps in a class II biosafety hood.
2. Begin to monitor parasitemia beginning at day 3 p.i., via blood smears. When the parasitemia is approximately 1–4 %, prepare to collect blood from infected mice.
3. Prepare a 50 mL polypropylene conical tube, containing 25 mL of RPMI/PS and 25 μL of heparin.
4. Euthanize all mice in accordance to the institutional ethics approval and harvest blood by cardiac puncture (*see* **Note 4**).
5. Once all blood has been collected, bring the volume up to 50 mL with RPMI/PS and centrifuge at 1,127 × *g* for 10 min at room temperature.
6. Carefully (because the blood cell pellet is loose) aspirate supernatant using a Pasteur pipette or other means, and estimate PCV by eye.
7. Add 2× PCV of freezing medium, drop-wise, while swirling over ice.
8. Aliquot 250–300 μL into labeled 1 mL cryo NUNC vials and transfer to a freezing container at room temperature. The freezing container should contain the correct volume of isopropanol (−1°/min). Place the container at −80 °C overnight.
9. The following day, transfer vials to long-term storage at −80 °C or liquid nitrogen.

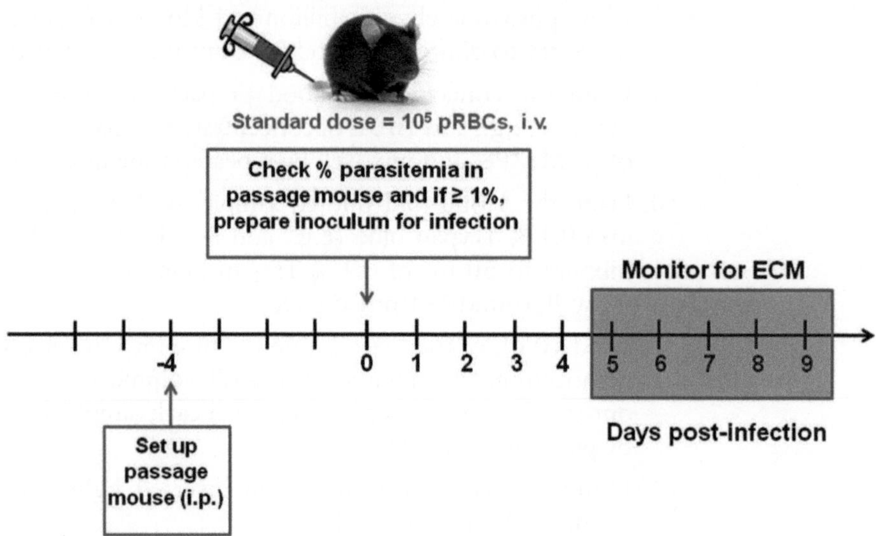

Fig. 2 Timeline of PbA infection. PbA parasites are passaged in vivo 4 days prior to infection (D-4). On the day of infection (day 0) mice are administered a standard dose of 10^5 parasitized red blood cells (pRBCs), intravenously (i.v.). Beginning at day 5 p.i. (120 h p.i.) mice are monitored twice daily for clinical signs of ECM

3.5 Setting Up PbA Infection in Mice

1. Thaw PbA stabilate (prepared in Protocol 3.4) and inject i.p. into a single C57BL/6J mouse.
2. Approximately 3–5 days later, assess parasitemia in the passage mouse via blood smear, and when it reaches 1–4 %, euthanize the passage mouse in accordance with the institutional ethics approval. Harvest blood by cardiac puncture.
3. Follow procedures outlined in Protocol 3.3 and i.v. inject 200 μL into the desired number of mice.
4. Monitor mice for clinical signs of experimental cerebral malaria (ECM) in accordance with ethics approval (Fig. 2).

3.6 Disease Assessment to Monitor Clinical ECM

1. Monitor mice twice daily from day 5 p.i., or when parasitemias exceed 4 % (*see* **Note 5**).
2. Assign ECM clinical scores according to the following symptoms: ruffled fur, hunching, wobbly gait, limb paralysis, convulsions, and coma. Each symptom is assigned a score of 1. Mice with a cumulative score of ≥4 should be euthanized by CO_2 asphyxiation, cervical dislocation, or other methods in accordance with ethics approval. A score of 5 should be assigned at the next time point, to denote death (Table 1 and Fig. 3).

3.7 Waste Management and Disposal

Disposable waste should be discarded in the autoclave waste containers. Liquid waste should be treated with 1 % Biodyne and left to sit for a minimum of 30 min prior to disposal down the sink with plenty of water.

Table 1
ECM clinical scoring system

Symptom	Score	Day p.i.
Ruffled fur	1	5
Hunching	1	5
Wobbly gait	1	6
Limb paralysis	1	6
Convulsions	1	6–7
Coma	1	6–7

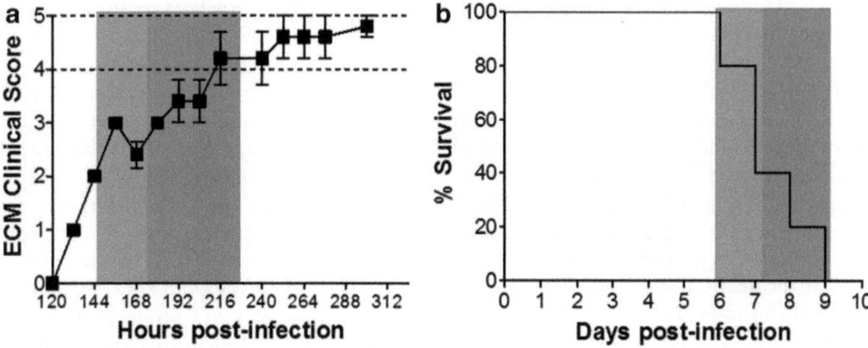

Fig. 3 Monitoring ECM and survival. Five C57BL/6J PbA-infected mice with a dose of 10^5 pRBCs i.v. were monitored for clinical signs of ECM (**a**) and survival (**b**) in accordance with standard scoring system and ethics approval, beginning at day 5 p.i. (120 h p.i.)

4 Notes

1. When staining glass slides, ensure that the glass surface (not the label) is completely immersed in the stain, by soaking the slide in and out a number of times with a pair of tweezers.
2. When transferring blood from the insulin syringe to the 10 mL tube (containing 5 mL media + 5 μL of heparin), ensure to push the plunger on the syringe gently, to reduce the risk of lysing red blood cells.
3. Avoid leaving inoculum at room temperature for long periods of time. However, if unavoidable, place on ice. When preparing the inoculum it is best to work quickly so that handling time is minimized.
4. The optimal volume of blood to collect from each mouse ranges from 500 to 800 μL. However, if all 20 mice are euthanized at one time, it will be difficult to obtain sufficient blood.

Therefore, euthanize in groups of 4–5 mice at any one time. Additionally, once the blood has been added to the 50 mL tube, gently invert the tube several times to ensure that the blood is mixed well with the RPMI/PS/heparin media, to prevent any clotting.

5. It is important to note that other clinical scoring systems have been reported, and these should also be considered as potential methods for assessing PbA-infected mice.

References

1. Engwerda CE, Belnoue E, Gruner AC, Renia L (2005) Experimental models of cerebral malaria. Curr Top Microbiol Immunol 297:103–143
2. Stevenson MM, Riley EM (2004) Innate immunity to malaria. Nat Rev Immunol 4(3): 169–180
3. Taylor-Robinson AW (2010) Regulation of immunity to Plasmodium: implications from mouse models for blood stage malaria vaccine design. Exp Parasitol 126(3):406–414
4. Langhorne J, Quin SJ, Sanni LA (2002) Mouse models of blood-stage malaria infections: immune responses and cytokines involved in protection and pathology. Chem Immunol 80(80):204–228
5. Brian de Souza J, Hafalla JC, Riley EM, Couper KN (2010) Cerebral malaria: why experimental murine models are required to understand the pathogenesis of disease. Parasitology 137(05):755–772
6. Hall N, Karras M, Raine JD et al (2005) A comprehensive survey of the Plasmodium life cycle by genomic, transcriptomic, and proteomic analyses. Science 307(5706):82–86
7. van Dijk MR, Waters AP, Janse CJ (1995) Stable transfection of malaria parasite blood stages. Science 268(5215):1358–1362
8. Tomas AM, van der Wel AM, Thomas AW, Janse CJ, Waters AP (1998) Transfection systems for animal models of malaria. Parasitol Today 14(6):245–249
9. Stevenson MM, Gros P, Olivier M, Fortin A, Serghides L (2010) Cerebral malaria: human versus mouse studies. Trends Parasitol 26(6):274–275
10. Amante FH, Haque A, Stanley AC et al (2010) Immune-mediated mechanisms of parasite tissue sequestration during experimental cerebral malaria. J Immunol 185(6):3632–3642
11. Baptista FG, Pamplona A, Pena AC, Mota MM, Pied S, Vigario AM (2010) Accumulation of Plasmodium berghei-infected red blood cells in the brain is crucial for the development of cerebral malaria in mice. Infect Immun 78(9):4033–4039
12. Schofield L, Grau GE (2005) Immunological processes in malaria pathogenesis. Nat Rev Immunol 5(9):722–735
13. Reis PA, Comim CM, Hermani F et al (2010) Cognitive dysfunction is sustained after rescue therapy in experimental cerebral malaria, and is reduced by additive antioxidant therapy. PLoS Pathog 6(6):e1000963
14. Desruisseaux MS, Gulinello M, Smith DN et al (2008) Cognitive dysfunction in mice infected with Plasmodium berghei strain ANKA. J Infect Dis 197(11):1621–1627
15. Thumwood CM, Hunt NH, Cowden WB, Clark IA (1988) Breakdown of the blood-brain barrier in murine cerebral malaria. Parasitology 96(03):579–589
16. Etienne-Manneville S, Manneville JB, Adamson P, Wilbourn B, Greenwood J, Couraud PO (2000) ICAM-1-coupled cytoskeletal rearrangements and transendothelial lymphocyte migration involve intracellular calcium signaling in brain endothelial cell lines. J Immunol 165(6):3375–3383
17. Haque A, Best SE, Unosson K et al (2011) Granzyme B expression by CD8+ T cells is required for the development of experimental cerebral malaria. J Immunol 186(11): 6148–6156
18. Nitcheu J, Bonduelle O, Combadiere C et al (2003) Perforin-dependent brain-infiltrating cytotoxic CD8+ T lymphocytes mediate experimental cerebral malaria pathogenesis. J Immunol 170(4):2221–2228
19. Potter S, Chan-Ling T, Ball HJ et al (2006) Perforin mediated apoptosis of cerebral microvascular endothelial cells during experimental cerebral malaria. Int J Parasitol 36(4): 485–496
20. Belnoue E, Kayibanda M, Vigario AM et al (2002) On the pathogenic role of

brain-sequestered αβ CD8+ T cells in experimental cerebral malaria. J Immunol 169(11): 6369–6375

21. Lovegrove FE, Gharib SA, Pena-Castillo L et al (2008) Parasite burden and CD36-mediated sequestration are determinants of acute lung injury in an experimental malaria model. PLoS Pathog 4(5):e1000068
22. Epiphanio S, Campos MG, Pamplona A et al (2010) VEGF promotes malaria-associated acute lung injury in mice. PLoS Pathog 6(5):e1000916
23. Helegbe G, Yanagi T, Senba M et al (2011) Histopathological studies in two strains of semi-immune mice infected with Plasmodium berghei ANKA after chronic exposure. Parasitol Res 108(4):807–814
24. Chang W-L, Jones SP, Lefer DJ et al (2001) CD8+-T-cell depletion ameliorates circulatory shock in Plasmodium berghei-infected mice. Infect Immun 69(12):7341–7348
25. Weerasinghe K, Galappaththy G, Fernando WP et al (2002) A safety and efficacy trial of artesunate, sulphadoxine-pyrimethamine and primaquine in P falciparum malaria. Ceylon Med J 47(3):83
26. Haque A, Best SE, Amante FH et al (2011) High parasite burdens cause liver damage in mice following Plasmodium berghei ANKA infection independently of CD8+ T cell-mediated immune pathology. Infect Immun 79(5):1882–1888
27. Berendt AR, Tumer GDH, Newbold CI (1994) Cerebral malaria: the sequestration hypothesis. Parasitol Today 10(10):412–414
28. MacPherson G, Warrell MJ, White NJ, Looareesuwan S, Warrell DA (1985) Human cerebral malaria. A quantitative ultrastructural analysis of parasitised erythrocyte sequestration. Am J Pathol 119:385–401
29. Dondorp AM, Desakorn V, Pongtavornpinyo W et al (2005) Estimation of the total parasite biomass in acute falciparum malaria from plasma PfHRP2. PLoS Med 2(8):e204
30. Fonager J, Pasini EM, Braks JA et al (2012) Reduced CD36-dependent tissue sequestration of Plasmodium-infected erythrocytes is detrimental to malaria parasite growth in vivo. J Exp Med 209(1):93–107
31. Nie CQ, Bernard NJ, Schofield L, Hansen DS (2007) CD4+ CD25+ regulatory T cells suppress CD4+ T-cell function and inhibit the development of Plasmodium berghei-specific TH1 responses involved in cerebral malaria pathogenesis. Infect Immun 75(5):2275–2282
32. Villegas-Mendez A, de Souza JB, Murungi L et al (2011) Heterogeneous and tissue-specific regulation of effector T cell responses by IFN-γ during Plasmodium berghei ANKA infection. J Immunol 187(6):2885–2897

Chapter 24

Characterization of HIV-1 Infection in the Humanized $Rag2^{-/-}\gamma c^{-/-}$ Mouse Model

Freddy M. Sanchez and Bradford K. Berges

Abstract

Engraftment of immunodeficient mice with a human immune system (humanized mice) provides a model system to study pathogens that target human immune cells. Humanized $Rag2^{-/-}\gamma c^{-/-}$ mice produce the major target cells of HIV-1 and these cells can be detected in primary and secondary lymphoid tissues, as well as in the vaginal and rectal mucosa and brain tissues. This humanized model has already yielded important findings on HIV-1 transmission, mechanisms of pathogenesis, and testing of novel antiviral strategies in vivo. Here, we describe the methods used to infect humanized mice with HIV-1 and to characterize plasma viral load and blood $CD4^+$ T cell depletion.

Key words Humanized mice, RAG-hu mice, Animal disease models, Hematopoietic stem cells, Stem cell transplantation, SCID-hu mice, BLT mice, HIV, HIV-1, AIDS

1 Introduction

HIV-1 is highly specific to infecting cells of human origin. Primary human cells and cell lines can be cultured and infected with HIV-1, and much knowledge has been gained about virus replication cycles, cellular pathogenesis, and antiviral drugs as a result. However, there is still much to be learned about HIV-1 pathogenesis and immune responses that cannot be studied in cultured cells. Specifically, living organisms are required for infection because of the diversity of cell types in the whole animal. Likewise, living organisms are capable of mounting immune responses to the virus in order to study virus–host interactions. Although SIV infection in nonhuman primates has been used as a model to study HIV-1 infection in humans, the differences in genetics between both viruses and hosts are problematic for translating those findings directly to HIV-1 in humans. For example, differences in host HLA genes are an obstacle to vaccine studies, and differences in viral genes and/or gene sequences have an impact on pathogenesis.

Irving C. Allen (ed.), *Mouse Models of Innate Immunity: Methods and Protocols*, Methods in Molecular Biology, vol. 1031, DOI 10.1007/978-1-62703-481-4_24, © Springer Science+Business Media, LLC 2013

Humanized mice are an exciting tool to study HIV-1 in vivo because they contain human HIV-1 target cells and can readily be infected with HIV-1. Humanized mice have been used to study HIV-1 for over 20 years [1–3]. The newer types of humanized mice are more profoundly immunodeficient than the original SCID mice and are also engrafted with human hematopoietic stem cells, resulting in enhanced engraftment as measured by total number of human cells, diversity of cell types, and distribution and duration of the graft [4, 5]. Human immune cells can be detected in a variety of lymphoid and non-lymphoid organs, and primary human adaptive immune responses (cellular and humoral) to HIV-1 and other pathogens are detectable [6]. Upon challenge with HIV-1 by either direct injection or mucosal routes, humanized mice become infected and viremia can be readily detected and quantified [7, 8]. Virus replication is detected in lymphoid and non-lymphoid organs, including brain tissue [9, 10]. Further, $CD4^+$ T cell depletion (the hallmark of AIDS) takes place in both blood and lymphoid organs [8, 11], and animals are responsive to various types of antiretroviral drugs [12]. HIV-1 produces a chronic infection in humanized mice, as in humans [13]. Diverse areas such as virus evolution, vaccine testing, gene therapy, and exploration of various types of pathogenesis are now being explored using the humanized mouse platform [1].

In this chapter we describe methods used to infect humanized mice with HIV-1. We also detail techniques used to measure plasma viral load via quantitative RT-PCR, and methods to quantify and track $CD4^+$ T cell depletion in peripheral blood samples.

2 Materials

2.1 HIV-1 Infection of Humanized $Rag2^{-/-}\gamma c^{-/-}$ Mice

1. Biohazard level 2 safety cabinet.
2. 8–10-week post-transplanted $Rag2^{-/-}\gamma c^{-/-}$ mice.
3. HIV-1 inoculum.
4. Complete DMEM medium with 10 % fetal bovine serum and 1× penicillin/streptomycin.
5. 1-cm^3 tuberculin syringes with 25-G × 5/8-in. needle.

2.2 Quantitative RT-PCR Analysis for Plasma Viral Load

1. Non-heparinized capillary tubes.
2. RNA isolation kit.
3. Sterile RNase-free pipette tips and EDTA-treated microfuge tubes.
4. DEPC-treated H_2O/nuclease-free H_2O.
5. Absolute ethanol (96–100 %).
6. HIV-1-specific PCR primers and TaqMan probe.
7. cDNA reverse transcription kit.

8. PCR tubes.
9. Microcentrifuge.
10. Vortex.
11. Thermal cycler.

2.3 Flow Cytometry for the Evaluation of Human CD4+ T Cell Levels

1. Peripheral blood collected from mouse tail vein.
2. EDTA-treated microcentrifuge tubes.
3. 10× ammonium chloride erythrocyte lysing solution: Dissolve 89.9 g of NH_4Cl, 10.0 g of $KHCO_3$, and 370.0 mg of tetrasodium EDTA in 1 l of ddH_2O. Adjust pH to 7.3. Store at 4 °C in full, tightly closed 50 ml tubes. Prior to use, dilute to 1× with ddH_2O and use immediately.
4. FACS staining buffer: 1× PBS, 0.1 % BSA, and 0.1 % sodium azide. Store at 4 °C.
5. 1× PBS.
6. Affinity purified human Fc receptor binding solution. Human Gamma Globulin (Jackson Immunoresearch Labs, West Grove, PA, USA), Normal Mouse Serum (Jackson Immunoresearch Labs), 2.4G2 monoclonal antibody to murine CD16/CD32 (BD, Franklin Lakes, NJ, USA). Reconstitute Normal Mouse Serum with 5.0 ml of ddH_2O. Add 2 ml of Human Gamma Globulin. Add 200 μl of 2.4G2 anti-mouse CD16/CD32. Store at 4 °C.
7. Species-specific antibodies for the pan-leukocyte marker CD45: hCD45-PE and mCD45-PE-Cy7 (eBioscience, San Diego, CA, USA).
8. Anti-human CD3 (BioLegend, clone HIT3a, PECy5, 6.25 μg/ml) and CD4 (eBioscience, clone RPA-T4, PECy7, 0.1 μg/μl) conjugated antibodies.
9. 1 % paraformaldehyde in 1× PBS: Paraformaldehyde does not dissolve effectively in PBS. Prepare a stock of 2 % paraformaldehyde in ddH_2O and a stock of 2× PBS in ddH_2O. Mix these solutions together in equal parts and store at 4 °C.
10. 12×75 mm, 5 ml polystyrene round-bottom tubes for flow cytometric analysis.
11. Microcentrifuge.

3 Methods

3.1 HIV-1 Infection of Humanized Rag2$^{-/-}\gamma c^{-/-}$ Mice

1. Prior to infection, mice are monitored for levels of human cell engraftment [6]. It is recommended to infect animals with at least 50 % of engraftment, and at least 8–10 weeks post reconstitution. Institutional approval to work with animals and HIV-1 must be sought prior to initiation of these studies (*see* **Note 1**).

2. To facilitate inoculation of animals, hold and restrain mice accordingly (*see* **Note 1**).
3. Mice are infected by either intraperitoneal or intravenous injection, using 1-cm^3 tuberculin syringes. HIV-1 inoculum is administered in a volume of 0.2 ml, in a dose that can range between 10^2 $TCID_{50}$ and 2×10^6 $TCID_{50}$. For a review of the different isolates and molecular clones of HIV-1 used for infection of humanized mice, *see* ref. 1. In our laboratory, we infect Rag2$^{-/-}\gamma c^{-/-}$ mice in the peritoneal cavity with 1×10^4 $TCID_{50}$ of HIV-$1_{Ba\text{-}L}$. This HIV-1 stock was obtained from Suzanne Gartner, Mikulas Popovic, and Robert Gallo through the AIDS Research and Reference Reagent Program Division [14].
4. Control animals are mock infected using 0.2 ml of complete DMEM.

3.2 Quantitative RT-PCR Analysis for Plasma Viral Load

1. Inside the hood, place the mouse to be sampled in a rodent restrainer. Pre-warming mice allows for collection of larger blood volumes (*see* **Note 2**). Carefully clean the tail with an alcohol-soaked cotton pad and allow drying. Hold the tail in a way that the veins can be easily located and cut for tail nick bleeding.
2. Using a clean surgical blade, make a small cut on the tail and immediately collect the blood into non-heparinized capillary tubes. Two capillary tubes (approximately 140 μl of blood) are sufficient to obtain plasma (for viral load) and blood cells (for $CD4^+$ T cell counts) from a single blood sample (*see* **Note 2**).
3. Expel the blood from the capillary tube into an RNase-free, EDTA-treated microfuge tube (*see* **Note 2**). Store samples on wet ice until RNA extraction. With a clean gauze pad, apply gentle pressure to the wound to stop bleeding and apply styptic powder to promote clotting. Return the animal to its cage.
4. Separate the cellular and plasma fractions by centrifugation at $900 \times g$ for 5 min.
5. Using barrier tips, separate plasma and blood cells into separate RNase-free microfuge tubes. If RNA extraction will be on a different day, store plasma at −80 °C. If RNA is extracted but reverse transcription will be performed at a later time, store extracted RNA at −80 °C.
6. RNA extraction, reverse transcription, and quantitative PCR can be performed with any of the commercially available kits by following the manufacturer's recommendations/protocols. The following list of primer and probe sequences are used in our laboratory for the production of cDNA and quantitative PCR specific for the HIV-1 LTR sequence [15]: *Forward primer*, 5-GCCTCAATAAAGCTTGCCTTGA-3; *Reverse*

primer, 5-GGCGCCACTGCTAGAGATTTT-3; *TaqMan probe*, 5-AAGTAGTGTGTGCCCGTCTGTTRTKTGACT-3 (FAM dye).

The cycling conditions are as follows: 30 min at 48 °C; 10 min at 95 °C; and 50 cycles of 95 °C for 15 s and 60 °C for 1 min.

7. Quantitation of viral load is performed by first calculating the copy number using the results of the quantitative PCR reaction to measure levels of viral cDNA. DNA samples with known copy number are used to calculate copy number of unknown samples, as described. Several additional factors need to be included when calculating the viral load in viral RNA copies/ml plasma (*see* **Note 3**).

3.3 Flow Cytometry for the Evaluation of Human CD4+ T Cell Levels in Peripheral Blood

1. Whole blood is collected as previously described in Subheading 3.2.
2. Remove red blood cells by lysis. Add 1.4 ml of 1× lysis buffer per 0.1 ml of mouse blood.
3. Incubate samples for 3–5 min at room temperature. Then centrifuge at 900×*g* for 5 min at room temperature.
4. Carefully aspirate and discard the supernatant, and resuspend the pellet in 0.8 ml of cold 1× PBS.
5. Centrifuge at 900×*g* for 5 min at room temperature. Aspirate and dispose of the supernatant. Resuspend the cell pellet in 0.1 ml of cold FACS staining buffer.
6. Before staining cells with FACS antibodies, pre-incubate the samples for 20 min on ice with 5 μl of human FcγR binding inhibitor. This will block nonspecific interaction of conjugated antibodies with Fc receptors on lymphocytes (*see* **Note 3**).
7. Stain peripheral blood cells with 3 μl each of hCD45-, hCD3-, and hCD4-conjugated antibodies. Mix gently and incubate samples on ice or at 4 °C in the dark for at least 30 min.
8. At this point, cells must be fixed to neutralize infectious agents (*see* **Note 1**). Also, fixation will preserve the samples if FACS analysis is planned for a different time. Fix the samples by adding 0.8 ml of 1 % paraformaldehyde in 1× PBS. If FACS analysis is to follow immediately, centrifuge samples at 900×*g* for 3 min at room temperature.
9. Discard supernatant and resuspend stained cells in 0.15 ml of 1× PBS. Pipet samples up and down until no clumps are present.
10. Transfer stained cells to 12×75 mm, 5 ml polystyrene round-bottom tubes, and proceed to analyze data on a flow cytometer (*see* **Notes 4–6**). Keep samples dark as much as possible to preserve signal intensity.

4 Notes

1. Extreme care must be taken when infecting animals with HIV-1 in order to prevent laboratory personnel exposure. All work with infectious HIV-1 must be performed inside a BSL-2^+ rated laminar flow hood. Animals must first be administered anesthesia (isoflurane) in order to prevent accidental puncture wounds. In addition, blood draws from HIV-1^+ animals are another possible source of exposure to lab workers. Infected blood samples intended for FACS analysis must be adequately fixed/inactivated prior to running through the flow cytometer in order to prevent exposure to the cytometer operator. All animal studies involving mice must first receive approval from the Institutional Animal Care and Use Committee prior to initiation. In addition, permission from the Institutional Biosafety Committee must be sought to work with HIV-1.
2. We commonly use a single blood draw to evaluate both viremia (Q-RT-PCR) and $CD4^+$ T cell counts (FACS analysis). Placing mouse cages onto a heating pad allows for greater volumes of blood to be collected. In order to prevent coagulation that will interfere with cellular analyses, anticoagulants must be used. We have found that heparin, which is a common anticoagulant, is an inhibitor of some types of PCR. Thus, we use untreated capillary tubes and quickly expel the blood into RNase-free, EDTA-treated microfuge tubes (EDTA is also an anticoagulant).
3. Viral load in humans is typically reported in viral RNA copies per milliliter of plasma, but mouse blood draws are typically restricted to ~150 μl of whole blood by animal care and use protocols. Thus, the size of plasma samples must be standardized or recorded for each individual sample. 50 μl of plasma can usually be obtained from each blood draw. In this case, samples must be normalized back to 1 ml by multiplying the final viral load by 20 because 1/20th of 1 ml of blood was used to extract viral RNA. Also, in most cases only a fraction of extracted RNA can be used for cDNA synthesis and quantitative PCR (note that one-step Q-RT-PCR kits are available). To account for only a fraction of RNA used for quantitation, one must also calculate for the fraction not measured by quantitative PCR. Due to these variables, a relatively high limit of detection is achieved despite the fact that quantitative PCR assays can typically detect below five copies of RNA. The following is an example calculation of viral load from raw data: 50 μl of plasma for RNA extraction = 1/20th of 1 ml of plasma; 10 μl of RNA (of 50 μl extracted) used for reverse transcription = 1/5th of RNA used; 5 μl of cDNA (out of 20 μl) for quantitative

PCR = 1/4th of cDNA used; thus, $20 \times 5 \times 4 = 400$ normalization factor. The viral load detected by quantitative PCR must be normalized by $20 \times 5 \times 4$ to determine viral load in RNA copies/1 ml of plasma.

4. FACS staining of immune cells adds an additional level of complexity due to cells that express the Fc receptor, which can bind antibodies by the constant, rather than the variable region. Humanized mouse blood samples are even more complicated because Fc receptor-bearing cells are present from two species in the same sample. We perform initial workup experiments with FACS antibodies on pure mouse blood or pure human blood to verify accuracy in staining. We block nonspecific staining by using a combination mouse/human Fc block consisting of anti-mouse CD16/CD32, human gamma globulin, and normal mouse serum (*see* Subheading 2). We typically use mouse monoclonal antibodies for FACS staining and we rarely detect background or cross-species staining.
5. Blood samples taken from a mouse are very small, and the number of human leukocytes is also smaller than an equivalent volume of human blood because engraftment does not reach normal human levels. In addition, there is variability in the engraftment rates from mouse to mouse and in the basal CD4$^+$-to-CD8$^+$ cell ratio in blood prior to infection. Thus, absolute CD4$^+$ T cell counts per volume of blood are not used to measure AIDS progression in humanized mice as is common in humans. CD4$^+$ T cell depletion in humanized mice is typically measured by calculating the ratio of CD4$^+$ T cells out of the total CD3$^+$ population, or alternatively by measuring the (CD4$^+$ cells)/(CD4$^+$ cells added to CD8$^+$ cells). In this way, a baseline CD4$^+$ ratio can be established for individual mice and then changes in the ratio can be readily calculated after HIV-1 infection.
6. HIV-1 pathogenesis is often more rapid and severe in humanized mice as compared to humans, especially when using CXCR4-tropic HIV-1. The reasons for this finding are not entirely clear, but one possible explanation is that the human antiviral immune response present in humanized mice to combat HIV-1 is thought to be relatively weak.

Acknowledgment

This work was supported by a Mentoring Environment Grant from Brigham Young University.

References

1. Berges BK, Rowan MR (2011) The utility of the new generation of humanized mice to study HIV-1 infection: transmission, prevention, pathogenesis, and treatment. Retrovirology 8:65
2. Mosier DE (1996) Human immunodeficiency virus infection of human cells transplanted to severe combined immunodeficient mice. Adv Immunol 63:79–125
3. Jamieson BD, Aldrovandi GM, Zack JA (1996) The SCID-hu mouse: an in-vivo model for HIV-1 pathogenesis and stem cell gene therapy for AIDS. Semin Immunol 8:215–221
4. Shultz LD, Ishikawa F, Greiner DL (2007) Humanized mice in translational biomedical research. Nat Rev Immunol 7:118–130
5. Legrand N, Ploss A, Balling R, Becker PD, Borsotti C, Brezillon N, Debarry J, de Jong Y, Deng H, Di Santo JP, Eisenbarth S, Eynon E, Flavell RA, Guzman CA, Huntington ND, Kremsdorf D, Manns MP, Manz MG, Mention JJ, Ott M, Rathinam C, Rice CM, Rongvaux A, Stevens S, Spits H, Strick-Marchand H, Takizawa H, van Lent AU, Wang C, Weijer K, Willinger T, Ziegler P (2009) Humanized mice for modeling human infectious disease: challenges, progress, and outlook. Cell Host Microbe 6:5–9
6. Traggiai E, Chicha L, Mazzucchelli L, Bronz L, Piffaretti JC, Lanzavecchia A, Manz MG (2004) Development of a human adaptive immune system in cord blood cell-transplanted mice. Science 304:104–107
7. Berges BK, Wheat WH, Palmer B, Connick E, Akkina R (2006) HIV-1 infection and CD4 T cell depletion in the humanized Rag2-/-gc-/- (RAG-hu) mouse model. Retrovirology 3:76
8. Baenziger S, Tussiwand R, Schlaepfer E, Mazzucchelli L, Heikenwalder M, Kurrer MO, Behnke S, Frey J, Oxenius A, Joller H, Aguzzi A, Manz MG, Speck RF (2006) Disseminated and sustained HIV infection in CD34+ cord blood cell-transplanted Rag2-/-gc-/- mice. Proc Natl Acad Sci U S A 103:15951–15956
9. Gorantla S, Makarov E, Finke-Dwyer J, Castanedo A, Holguin A, Gebhart CL, Gendelman HE, Poluektova L (2011) Links between progressive HIV-1 infection of humanized mice and viral neuropathogenesis. Am J Pathol 177:2938–2949
10. Dash PK, Gorantla S, Gendelman HE, Knibbe J, Casale GP, Makarov E, Epstein AA, Gelbard HA, Boska MD, Poluektova LY (2011) Loss of neuronal integrity during progressive HIV-1 infection of humanized mice. J Neurosci 31:3148–3157
11. Berges BK, Akkina SR, Folkvord JM, Connick E, Akkina R (2008) Mucosal transmission of R5 and X4 tropic HIV-1 via vaginal and rectal routes in humanized Rag2-/-gc-/- (RAG-hu) mice. Virology 373:342–351
12. Choudhary SK, Rezk NL, Ince WL, Cheema M, Zhang L, Su L, Swanstrom R, Kashuba AD, Margolis DM (2009) Suppression of HIV-1 viremia with reverse transcriptase and integrase inhibitors, CD4+ T cell recovery, and viral rebound upon therapy interruption in a new model for HIV treatment in the humanized Rag2-/- c-/- mice. J Virol 83: 8254–8258
13. Berges BK, Akkina SR, Remling L, Akkina R (2010) Humanized Rag2(-/-) gammac(-/-) (RAG-hu) mice can sustain long-term chronic HIV-1 infection lasting more than a year. Virology 397:100–103
14. Gartner S, Markovits P, Markovitz DM, Kaplan MH, Gallo RC, Popovic M (1986) The role of mononuclear phagocytes in HTLV-III/LAV infection. Science 233(4760):215–219
15. Rouet F, Ekouevi DK, Chaix ML, Burgard M, Inwoley A, Tony TD, Danel C, Anglaret X, Leroy V, Msellati P, Dabis F, Rouzioux C (2005) Transfer and evaluation of an automated, low-cost real-time reverse transcription-PCR test for diagnosis and monitoring of human immunodeficiency virus type 1 infection in a West African resource-limited setting. J Clin Microbiol 43:2709–2717

Index

Irving C. Allen (ed.), *Mouse Models of Innate Immunity: Methods and Protocols*, Methods in Molecular Biology, vol. 1031, DOI 10.1007/978-1-62703-481-4, © Springer Science+Business Media, LLC 2013

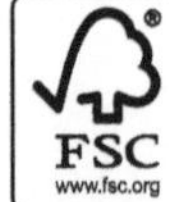

MIX
Papier aus verantwortungsvollen Quellen
Paper from responsible sources
FSC® C105338

If you have any concerns about our products,
you can contact us on
ProductSafety@springernature.com

In case Publisher is established outside the EU,
the EU authorized representative is:
Springer Nature Customer Service Center GmbH
Europaplatz 3, 69115 Heidelberg, Germany

Printed by Libri Plureos GmbH
in Hamburg, Germany